Mechatronics in Medicine

Mechatronics in Medicine

A Biomedical Engineering Approach

Siamak Najarian
Javad Dargahi
Goldis Darbemamieh
Siamak H. Farkoush

McGraw Hill

New York Chicago San Francisco
Lisbon London Madrid Mexico City
Milan New Delhi San Juan
Seoul Singapore Sydney Toronto

The McGraw-Hill Companies

Cataloging-in-Publication Data is on file with the Library of Congress.

Mechatronics in Medicine: A Biomedical Engineering Approach

1 2 3 4 5 6 7 8 9 0 LPI/LPI 1 9 8 7 6 5 4 3 2 1

ISBN 978-0-07-176896-2
MHID 0-07-176896-3

The pages within this book were printed on acid-free paper.

Sponsoring Editor
Michael Penn

Acquisitions Coordinator
Bridget Thoreson

Editorial Supervisor
David E. Fogarty

Project Manager
Ridhi Mathur,
Cenveo Publisher Services

Copy Editor
Pia Oberoi

Proofreader
Surendra Nath Shivam,
Cenveo Publisher Services

Production Supervisor
Pamela A. Pelton

Composition
Cenveo Publisher Services

Art Director, Cover
Jeff Weeks

About the Authors

Siamak Najarian serves as the Full-Professor of Biomedical Engineering at Amirkabir University of Technology. He has completed his Ph.D. in Biomedical Engineering at Oxford University, England and had a postdoctoral position at the same university for one year. His research interests are the applications of artificial tactile sensing (especially in robotic surgery), mechatronics in biological systems, and design of artificial organs. He is the author and translator of 26 books in the field of biomedical engineering, 9 of which are written in English. Prof. Najarian has published more than 170 international journal and conference papers in the field of biomedical engineering along with two international books in the same field. One of his books entitled *Artificial Tactile Sensing in Biomedical Engineering* achieved the rank of finalist at the 2009 PROSE Awards among all the entries in the Engineering and Technology category. He was the first author of the mentioned book published in 2009 by McGraw-Hill.

Javad Dargahi received his B.Sc. and M.Sc. degrees in Mechanical Engineering from University of Paisley, UK. He received his Ph.D. degree from Glasgow Caledonian University, Glasgow in the area of Robotic Tactile Sensing in 1993. He worked as an Assistant Professor in the Biomedical Engineering Department at Amirkabir University of Technology, Tehran in 1994. He was a Senior Post-Doctoral Research Fellow with the Micromachining/Medical Robotics Group at Simon Fraser University, Burnaby, in 1997. He worked as a full-time lecturer in the Mechanical Engineering Department at University of New Brunswick in 1999. Dr. Dargahi was employed in Pega Medical Company in Montreal, in 2001. He joined Concordia University, as an Assistant Professor in the Department of Mechanical and Industrial Engineering in 2001. He was promoted to Associate Professor and then Professor in 2006 and 2011. His research areas include micromechatronics in surgery, design and fabrication of haptic sensors and feedback systems for minimally invasive surgery and robotics, microfabrication of sensors and actuators, and telemanipulation in robotic surgery. Dr. Dargahi has published over 145 refereed journal and conference papers. He is the coauthor of a book *Artificial Tactile Sensing in Biomedical Engineering*, which was published by McGraw-Hill in 2009. This book was the runner-up in the Engineering & Technology category of the Association of American Publishers' Professional and Scholarly Excellence Awards. Dr. Dargahi has a patent entitled: "System for sensing and displaying force and softness." He has been a reviewer of several NASA proposals in the area of crew health and performance in a space exploration mission.

Goldis Darbemamieh received her B.Sc. degree in Mechanical Engineering from Isfahan University of Technology, Iran and her M.Sc. and Ph.D. degrees in Biomedical Engineering from Amirkabir University of Technology, Iran. Her M.Sc. thesis has been selected as the best M.Sc. thesis in the whole country (Iran) in the field of Engineering and Technology and the thesis has been published as a book. She has been also awarded as the best M.Sc. student of the country in 2009 for her enthusiastic and successful studies. Dr. Darbemamieh has published more than 15 international journal and conference papers, and her research interests are artificial tactile sensing, mechatronics, robotic surgery, and smart surgical instruments.

Siamak Hajizadeh Farkoush received his B.Sc. degree in Software Engineering from University of Science and Culture, Iran and his M.Sc. and Ph.D. degrees in Biomedical Engineering from Amirkabir University of Technology, Iran. His research interests are robotics, mechatronics, and smart surgical instruments and he has registered three patents in the European patent office in 2006 in these fields. Mr. Hajizadeh Farkoush has been awarded the silver medal in international competition of invention in the Geneva, Swiss in 2008 and has won the second prize in the Competition of Robocup 2006 in Bremen, Germany. He has won the first national prize in Robowar competition in Iran in 2003 and has been also awarded in Kharazmi International Festivals in 1998, 1999, and 2000 in Iran for his proposed robotic projects.

Contents

Preface

Mechatronics is a multidisciplinary field that, through an integrated design approach, makes synergistic use of mechanics, electronics, control theory, computer science, and information technology during the development of electromechanical systems and products. By referring to pertinent aspects contained in a number existing works published in the field of mechatronics, we have produced this unique book, *Mechatronics in Medicine: A Biomedical Engineering Approach*, which, for the first time, presents applications of mechatronics in the field of medicine from a biomedical engineering standpoint.

The authors of this book have longtime experience in different universities and research centers and are accredited with many publications and journals articles in the medical field. In addition to providing a basic overview of mechatronics, this book also provides a description of multidisciplinary medical systems which, hopefully, will provide engineers and physicians with an enlightened insight into the design and operation of such systems.

This book contains nine chapters, presenting practical and fundamental concepts in the field of mechatronics and its applications in medicine and biomedical engineering. Each chapter is arranged in such a way that the reader will become familiar with various components of a mechatronics system, step-by-step, both from the hardware and software points of view. Each chapter deals with some of the most recent medical mechatronics case studies in order to provide contemporary details of their design, operation, and applications. Some of the figures of the book will appear in color on the following Web site: www.mhprofessional.com/mmbea

The goals and main concepts provided in each chapter are as follows:

Chapter 1 introduces mechatronics and describes the architecture and basic components of a mechatronics system including its design concept, framework, and importance in medical applications.

Chapter 2 presents sensing technologies and their applications in mechatronics with a biomedical approach. Various sensors and transducers are explained with emphasis on the role of sensor technologies such as capacitance, inductance, Hall effect, resistance, piezoelectricity, light, and sound waves. Different characteristics of sensors such as transfer function, accuracy, resolution, calibration, hysteresis, and response time are also explained together with a compilation of the most commonly used and applicable sensors. Machine vision and its application in mechatronics are also discussed followed by a presentation of sensors that have specialized applications in the medical field.

Chapter 3 defines and explains electrical actuators and fluid/compressed gas power actuators, followed by a description of other types of actuators such as chemical, shape memory alloy, ionic polymer-metal composite, and MEMS. A brief description of feedback sensors and the criteria for actuator selection is also given in this chapter.

Chapter 4 deals with mechanisms and mechanical devices used in mechatronics systems including rack and pinions, gears, chains, belt drives, linkages, cams, etc. Different types of such devices, and their function, are explained and are classified in six categories according to their function, namely, conversion of rotational motion into linear motion and vice versa, changing rotational speed/torque and the angular orientation of rotational motion, transformation of rotary motion in one plane to another, brakes and clutches, creation of a particular manner of motion, and bearings.

Chapter 5 deals with the principles and methods of processing and controlling mechatronics systems and includes the basics of control, data acquisition, microprocessors, and microcontrollers.

Chapter 6 briefly describes the common tools and methods used in making mechatronics systems intelligent, especially those which are used in the field of medicine and biomedical engineering. Other main concepts discussed in this chapter are artificial intelligence, expert systems, artificial neural networks, fuzzy systems, and neuro fuzzy systems.

Chapter 7 covers the general basis and function of various medical imaging systems. Medical images are the source of valuable data with which a specialist can detect any abnormalities such as fractures, tumorous tissues, and signs of stenosis in the arteries. Also explained are high-tech medical devices in which mechatronics plays a significant and key role. Following this is a discussion on various medical imaging systems including medical ultrasound, MRI, CT scan, and nuclear imaging.

Chapter 8 details the most important applications of mechatronics in the medical and biomedical engineering fields including robotics in medicine, smart instruments and probes, and navigation.

Chapter 9 presents various medical mechatronics from actual case studies in which recently developed devices and techniques were used in varied fields of medical practice. These include handheld snake-like robots, smart-probes for detecting kidney stones and breast cancer, an ankle-sprain evaluation system, an active prosthetic knee, an instrument for esophagectomy and a smart-system for detecting cardiovascular plaque.

Siamak Najarian, *Full-Professor of Biomedical Engineering, Amirkabir University of Technology, Tehran, Iran*

Javad Dargahi, *Full-Professor of Mechanical Engineering, Concordia University, Montreal, Canada*

Goldis Darbemamieh, *Ph.D. in Biomedical Engineering, Amirkabir University of Technology, Tehran, Iran*

Siamak Hajizadeh Farkoush, *Ph.D. in Biomedical Engineering, Amirkabir University of Technology, Tehran, Iran*

Acknowledgments

The authors would like to thank the many people who have contributed to this book. They would also like to acknowledge, and offer their sincere appreciation to all individuals who have assisted them in this work and the organizational help provided by various institutes and companies who allowed the authors free use of their material.

The authors would like to give special thanks to Mr. Pedram Pahlavan (M.Sc. in Biomedical Engineering) for his valuable help in preparing this book and also to Mr. Arthur Couch for his excellent editing work on the book.

Mechatronics in Medicine

CHAPTER 1

Introduction to Mechatronics

1.1 Introduction

Because of the large number of technological advances that have recently been made in a wide variety of multidisciplinary fields, the boundary between engineering sciences and the relative applications to which they can be applied has become blurred.

Modern devices are being used in advanced mechanical, electrical, and computer systems for industrial applications, and to assist in research. For instance, a modern textile machine utilizing electronics and sensory control systems performs more efficiently than a machine using complicated mechanisms. Another example is the modern automotive industry in which automobiles now integrate mechanical functions with electronic controls in order to provide more advantages such as higher performance and lower fuel consumption.

Mechatronics is a multidisciplinary engineering field, the combination of mechanical engineering, electrical engineering, and software engineering. In this chapter, mechatronic systems are discussed, including their design concept, framework, and importance in medical applications.

1.2 Mechatronic Systems

The Yasakawa Electric Company in Japan coined the word "mechatronics" in 1969. In the 1970s and 1980s, research and development activities made way for the growth and evolution of mechatronics. Yasakawa defined *mechatronics* in trademark application documents as follows:[1,2] "The word, mechatronics, is composed of 'mecha' from mechanism and the 'tronics' from electronics. That is to say technologies and developed products will now incorporate electronics more intimately and organically into mechanisms, making it impossible to tell where one ends and the other begins."

After Yasakawa suggested the original definition for mechatronics, some other definitions were also presented as follows:[3] In 1996, Harashima, Tomizuka, and Fukuda defined mechatronics as being "the synergistic integration of mechanical engineering, with electronics and intelligent computer control in the design and manufacturing of industrial products and processes."[4] In the same year, Auslander and

Kempf suggested another definition of mechatronics as being "the application of complex decision making to the operation of physical systems."[5] In 1997, Shetty and Kolk defined mechatronics as "a methodology used for the optimal design of electromechanical products."[6] In his recent book on mechatronics, Bolton presented yet another definition by saying "a mechatronic system is not just a marriage of electrical and mechanical systems and is more than just a control system; the mechatronic system is a complete integration of them all."[7] Although all the preceding definitions of mechatronics are correct and accurate, not one of them is fully definitive since the field of mechatronics is still in its infancy.[3]

Up to the early part of the twentieth century, mechanical systems were primarily used, and it was not until the 1920s that electrical drives were incorporated into mechanical systems. Since 1935, mechanical systems equipped with automatic control were devised, and in the 1950s electromechanical systems were developed as a result of progress in control engineering. In the 1960s, digital computers and information technology were developed with the advent of advances in the integrated circuit (IC) and microprocessor technologies. In the mid-1970s mechanical systems with digital control were developed and products or processes were integrated with electronics. It was not until 1980 that electromechanical systems, which had hitherto consisted of separate electrical and mechanical parts, were replaced by integrated electronic-mechanical systems containing sensors, actuators, and digital microelectronics culminating in the formation of the mechatronic system.

By definition, *synergy* is the ability of a group to outperform even its best individual member. It can be said about mechatronics, that through an integrated design approach this system does make synergistic use of mechanics, electronics, control theory, computer science, and information technology in the development of electromechanical systems and products. This means that mechatronics is a multidisciplinary engineering field which consists of mechanical engineering, electronics and electrical engineering, software engineering used in manufacturing, medicine, and the service industries. The main disciplines of mechatronics are shown in Fig. 1.1.

A typical mechatronic system consists of sensors, transducers, actuators, mechanisms, mechanical components, data acquisition devices, processing and control systems, software and expert system. The components of a mechatronic system are shown in Fig. 1.2.

Examples of mechatronic systems include, but are not limited to, space technology, transportation, optical telecommunications, automobiles, microwaves, automated manufacturing plants, wireless network enabled devices, micro electromechanical systems

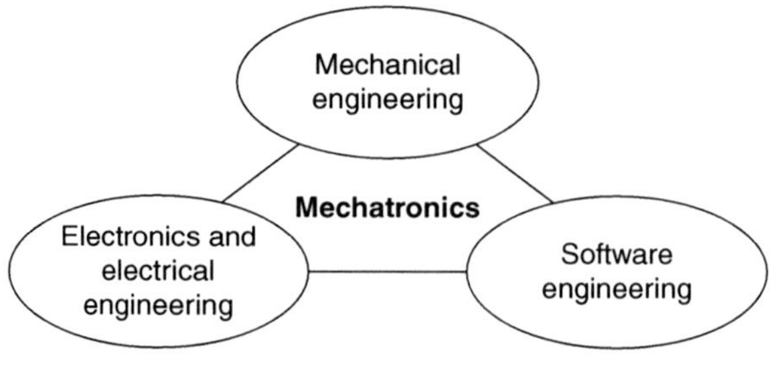

FIGURE 1.1 The main disciplines of mechatronics as a multidisciplinary engineering field.

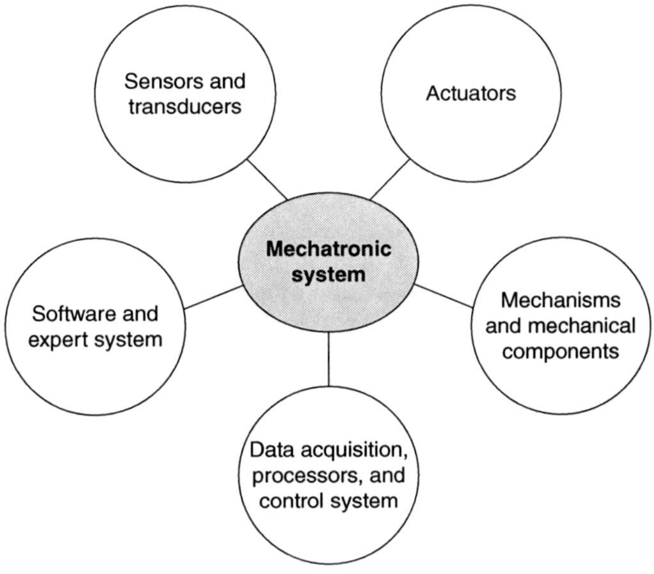

Figure 1.2 Components of a mechatronic system.

(MEMS), automated diagnostic systems, biomedical devices, surgical devices, robots, and artificial organs.

The Japanese Society for the Promotion of Machine Industry (JSPMI), in the late 1970s, categorized mechatronic systems and products into four main classes as follows:[1]

Class I: Primarily mechanical products incorporated with electronics to have enhanced functionality. Two examples of this are numerically controlled machine tools and variable speed drives in manufacturing machines.

Class II: Classical mechanical systems with significantly updated internal devices including electronics but with an unchanged external user interface. Two examples are the modern sewing machine and automated manufacturing systems.

Class III: Systems whose functionality is similar to the classical mechanical system, but their internal mechanisms are replaced by electronics. An example of this is the digital watch.

Class IV: Products designed with synergistic integration of mechanical and electronic technologies. Examples are photocopiers, intelligent washers and dryers, and automatic ovens.

The above mechatronics product classes are based on development in various technologies. Class I products were generated by using servo technology, power electronics, and control theory. Class II products were generated by using early computational and memory devices and custom circuit design capabilities. Class III products were based on the microprocessor and integrated circuits to replace mechanical systems, and Class IV products relied on the beginning of true mechatronic systems which were the combination of mechanical systems and electronics.[3]

In the classical development of an electromechanical system, the mechanical and electrical components are first designed or selected separately and then integrated with other hardware and software components. However, in the mechatronics approach, the whole electromechanical system is designed simultaneously in an integrated manner by a multidisciplinary team of professionals.

A system produced by interconnecting a set of separately designed and constructed components will not provide the same level of performance as a mechatronic system that employs an integrated approach for design, development, and execution. The main reason is that the best operation can only be achieved through an integrated approach to design, development, and execution by ensuring that optimum compatibility exists between each discrete entity in the system.

In general, a mechatronics product is more efficient, cost effective, compact, accurate, reliable, flexible and practical, and mechanically simpler than an alternative product.[8] Although by using a complex control system the performance of such an alternative system can be improved, it would require the additional cost of sensors, instrumentation, control hardware and software.[8]

1.3 Mechatronics Design Concept and Framework

Mechatronics design is a combination of physical modeling systems and simulation techniques. It is used to design complex machines by combining mechanical and physical characteristics with electronics and software to achieve a real-time prototype. In designing a mechatronic system, various factors such as quality, performance, cost, safety, speed, etc., must be considered and optimized.

One example of mechatronic systems is robot manipulation. The robotics industry came to the fore in the late 1970s and early 1980s due to the increasing availability of low-cost digital signal processors (DSPs) and microprocessors that possessed high-computational power. Robotic manipulators are used in many applications, such as manufacturing processes and robotic assisted surgery. A robotic manipulator has four major subsystems, and every modern mechatronic system has the same subsystem functionalities:[9]

1. A mechanism to transfer motion from an actuator to the instrument.
2. An actuator (a motor and power amplifier, a hydraulic cylinder and valve) and power source (DC power supply, internal combustion engine and pump).
3. Sensors to measure the motion variables.
4. A controller (data acquisition, microcontroller, microprocessor and DSPs) together with operator user interface devices and communication capabilities to other intelligent devices.

Because a mechatronic system usually consists of various types of interconnected components and elements, there is energy conversion from one form to another, especially between electrical energy and mechanical energy. In an electromechanical system, there is an interaction or coupling between the electrical dynamics and the mechanical dynamics in which each have an effect on the other. The dynamic coupling between various components of a system shows that it is more prudent to design the system as a whole rather than designing the electrical parts and the mechanical parts separately.

The following problems can occur when independently designed components are interconnected:[8]

1. The original characteristics and operating conditions of the components tend to change as a result of loading or dynamic interactions.
2. Perfect compatibility of two independently designed components will be practically impossible and a component is likely to become either underutilized or overloaded.
3. Some of the external variables in the components will become internal and hidden as a result of interconnection, which causes potential problems that cannot be explicitly monitored through sensing and, therefore, cannot be directly controlled.

The limitations inherent within most classical mechanical-electronic systems include: the lack of appropriate sensors and actuators, inadequate lifetime under rough operating conditions (acceleration, temperature, and contamination), large space requirements, bulky cabling, and relatively slow data processing.[3] In the design of a mechatronic system, however, with the advent of miniaturization, robustness, and computing power of microelectronic components, electronics can be improved and more autonomous systems can be visualized, such as capsuled units with touchless signal transfer or bus connections, and robust microelectronics.[3]

There are two types of integrations in a mechatronic system: the integration of components (hardware integration) and the integration of information processing (software integration).[3]

Hardware integration results from designing the mechatronic system as an overall system and inserting sensors, actuators, and microcomputers into the mechanical system. Integrated sensors and microcomputers form smart sensors, and integrated actuators and microcomputers form smart actuators. For larger systems, bus connections will replace cables and so there are several possibilities to generate an integrated overall system by proper integration of the hardware.[3] Software integration, or the integration of information processing, is generally based on advanced control functions. Besides a basic control, an additional influence may be caused by processing available signals at higher levels, including the solution of tasks such as fault diagnosis, optimization, and general process management. Therefore, a knowledge base that comprises methods for design and information gathering, process models, and performance criteria is required.[3]

1.4 Importance of Mechatronics in Medical Applications

Due to the high sensitivity of medical equipment, for which the hygienic aspect must be considered, rapid developments in facilitating and observing high standards of hygiene and treatment are always observed. These developments naturally require different specialties in order to design accurate, intelligent, and efficient systems. Medical instruments were always designed to fulfill a specific function and, in the right hands, were invariably used to good purpose. Introduction of modern devices and fields such as the artificial heart, robotic surgery, and intelligent probes shows that the efficiency of conventional tools depends as much on the appropriate combination of mechanics, electronics, and computer science as it does on the skilful use to which they are subsequently put. For instance, within the field of medicine, telerobotics is a complicated mechatronic system that can be used in minimally invasive surgeries to perform surgical procedures with a very high degree of precision. The design and development of telerobotic systems, therefore, plays an important role in improving the quality of surgical procedures and reducing potential problems. Using mechatronic systems, researchers are also investigating implantation techniques in the human body, using micro- and nanotechnology to repair or replace damaged physiological functions.

This book introduces and discusses modern solutions for utilizing mechatronics in designing these novel methods and optimizing conventional medical instruments. Because mechatronics fosters new concepts and development in an ever-increasing number of fields and disciplines, new devices will always be introduced, and advances made, that will spearhead and encourage further research. If this is so, mechatronics will surely have a bright and highly influential future.

References

1. N. Kyura and H. Oho. Mechatronics—An Industrial Perspective. *IEEE/ASME Transactions on Mechatronics,* vol. 1, no. 1, 1996, pp. 10–15.
2. T. Mori. Mechatronics Yasakawa Internal Trademark Application Memo 21.131.01, July 12, 1969.
3. R. H. Bishop (Ed.) *Mechatronics— An Introduction, CRC*-Taylor and Francis, 2006.
4. F. Harashima, M. Tomizuka, and T. Fukuda. Mechatronics—What Is It, Why, and How?—An Editorial. *IEEE/ASME Transactions on Mechatronics,* vol. 1, no. 1, 1996, pp. 1–4.
5. D. M. Auslander and C. J. Kempf. *Mechatronics: Mechanical System Interfacing,* Prentice-Hall, 1996.
6. D. Shetty and R. A. Kolk. *Mechatronic System Design,* PWS Publishing Company, 1997.
7. W. Bolton. *Mechatronics: Electrical Control Systems in Mechanical and Electrical Engineering,* 2nd ed., Addison-Wesley Longman, 1999.
8. C. W. De Silva. *Mechatronics: An Integrated Approach,* CRC Press, 2005.
9. S. Cetinkunt. *Mechatronics,* John Wiley & Sons, Inc., 2007.

CHAPTER 2
Sensing Technology

2.1 Introduction

In mechatronic systems, a great diversity of different parameters need to be measured including displacement, force, pressure, torque, temperature, flow, etc. These parameters are primary aspects in various fields such as electrical engineering, mechanical engineering, medicine, and biomedical engineering. All inputs to mechatronic systems come from various forms of sensory devices or communications from other systems.[1]

In this chapter, sensing technologies and their applications in mechatronics are discussed with a biomedical approach. In Sec. 2.2, sensors and transducers are discussed and explained with emphasis on the role of sensor technologies operating under the auspices of capacitance, inductance, Hall effect, resistance, piezoelectricity, light, and sound waves. Different characteristics of sensors such as transfer function, accuracy, resolution, calibration, hysteresis, and response time are also explained in this section together with a compilation of the most commonly used and applicable sensors. In Sec. 2.3, machine vision and its application in mechatronics is discussed and in Sec. 2.4, sensor applications in medicine are presented.

2.2 Transducers and Sensors

In general, a sensor is the complete assembly required to detect and communicate a particular event, while a transducer is the element within that assembly which accomplishes only the detection of the event. A transducer converts an input to an output that can be exploited to accomplish the sensing task. It is actuated by power from one system and supplies power, usually in another form, to a second system. For example, a thermocouple is a transducer that converts thermal energy into electrical energy; a loudspeaker is a transducer that converts electrical energy into acoustical energy. *Efficiency* is an important parameter in transducers and is defined as being the ratio of the energy output to the total energy input. Some energy is always dissipated during energy conversion so therefore no transducer is 100 percent efficient.

A sensor is a device that responds to a physical stimulus (such as heat, light, sound, pressure, magnetism, or a particular motion) and transmits a resulting impulse (as for measurement or operating a control). Most sensors propagate an electrical output signal and, on those occasions when they detect one form of energy and produce a signal in a different form of energy, they act as a transducer.[1] Sensors can be classified according to the conversion principle, the quantity being measured, the technology used, or the application.[2] Here, the specific application of a sensor determines its category. Sensors can be either passive or active. Passive sensors are self-generating sensors that generate the output signal directly and without the necessity of any external energy supply. An example of a passive sensor is the piezoelectric sensor in which a voltage is generated in proportion to an applied pressure. Conversely, active sensors are dynamically unable to produce an output signal until they are supplied with power from an external signal from a source other than that which is being sensed. An example of an active sensor is the strain gauge sensor whose electrical resistance changes in proportion to the strain applied. When used in a voltage divider circuit, the output voltage will vary in direct proportion to the change in resistance.

Sensors are also classified as being either absolute or relative. Absolute sensors detect a stimulus in reference to an absolute physical scale that is independent of the measurement conditions, whereas a relative sensor produces a signal that relates to some special case.[3] An example of absolute and relative sensors is the rotary encoder which is an electro-mechanical device that converts the angular position (or motion) of a shaft into either an analog or digital code. For this device, absolute sensing produces a unique digital code for each distinct angle of the shaft and, even if the shaft stops moving, its last angular position is saved; relative sensing keeps track of motion and can be used to determine position and velocity which can be either linear or rotary motion.

Sensors can also be classified to digital and analog sensors. Digital sensors produce discrete output signals that provide on/off results or stepped binary results. An example of an on/off digital sensor is the proximity switch and an example of a digital sensor with binary output is an encoder. The analog sensor, on the other hand, produces a continuous output signal and when the controller of the system is digital, an analog-to-digital (A/D) converter is needed to convert the analog signals into digital values. An example of an analog sensor is the potentiometer which provides a variable resistance.

2.2.1 Sensor Technologies

In order to detect and measure the physical properties of each type of sensor, various technologies can be used which, in themselves, have their own purpose and criteria. Sensor technology is mainly classified according to transduction principles and can be measured using more than one technology based on different transduction methods. For example, resistance, capacitance, and piezoelectric effect sensors can be used for measuring an applied force. Here, some of the most common principles of transduction used in mechatronics systems are discussed.

2.2.1.1 Capacitance

Any physical property that changes its capacitance can be measured by capacitive sensors. This transduction mechanism has many applications in mechatronics systems such as measuring displacement, velocity, acceleration, force, pressure, vacuum, flow, fluid level, audio sound field, and relative humidity.[4] For measuring a change in capacity of such a sensor, an electric circuit is required to convert this change into either a voltage or a frequency.[5] A capacitive sensor consists of two plates and a dielectric material between each plate as shown in Fig. 2.1.

Using a dielectric material between two plates to form a capacitor was first investigated by Michael Faraday in 1837. He discovered that having a dielectric material between the plates increases the capacitance of the sensor in proportion to the dielectric constant of the material.[3] In practice, most dielectric materials are solid and include porcelain (ceramic), mica, glass, plastics, and the oxides of various metals. Some liquids

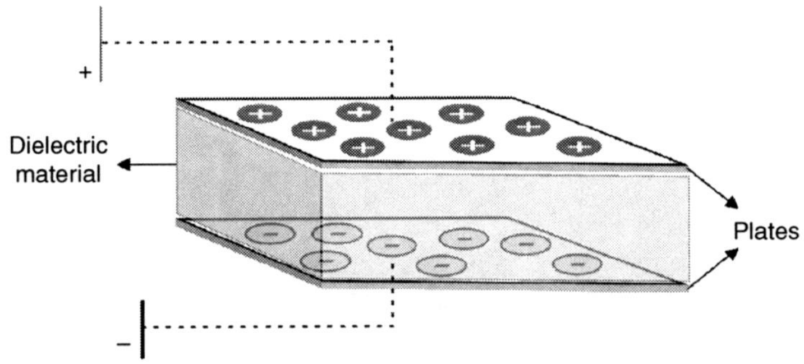

FIGURE 2.1 Schematic structure of a capacitive sensor.

and gases can also serve as good dielectric materials. Dry air is an excellent dielectric, and a vacuum is an exceptionally efficient dielectric. The capacitance of a parallel-plate capacitor C is given as shown in Eq. (2.1):

$$C = \frac{\varepsilon_0 \varepsilon_r A}{d} \tag{2.1}$$

where $\varepsilon_0 = 8.85 \times 10^{-12}$ F·m^{-1} is the permittivity of free space. ε_r is relative permittivity or dielectric constant of the dielectric material and $\varepsilon_r = 1$ for air.[4] A is the area of the plates and d is the distance between the plates. According to Eq. (2.1), the capacitance of a parallel-plate capacitor depends on the dielectric constant of the dielectric material, the area of the plates and the distance between the plates. The capacitance changes directly with the dielectric constant of the dielectric material and the area of the plates, but it changes inversely with the distance between the plates of the capacitor. For example, when an external force is applied to a capacitive sensor, the distance between the plates d is reduced and subsequently, the capacitance is increased. Therefore, any change in applied force will cause proportional changes in the capacitance. Capacitive sensors have many applications in industry and clinical fields and they can be used both in discrete and array types.[5]

2.2.1.2 Inductance

Inductance is derived from an inductor which is a wound coil within which a strong magnetic field is generated when current flows through it. Any physical property such as displacement, force, pressure, torque, vibration velocity, and acceleration that can change the self-inductance of a coil, or the common inductance of two coils, can be measured by an inductive sensor.[4] In 1831, both Michael Faraday in England and Joseph Henry in the United States discovered that a changing magnetic field induces electric current in a wire whereas a stationary magnetic field does not.[3] In inductive sensors, a physical phenomenon affects the reluctance of the magnetic field which, in turn, changes the induced electric current. An inductive sensor consists of a ferromagnetic core around which conducting wire is wound as shown in Fig. 2.2. When the core moves into the coil, the inductance increases and reaches its maximum when the core is in the middle of the coil.

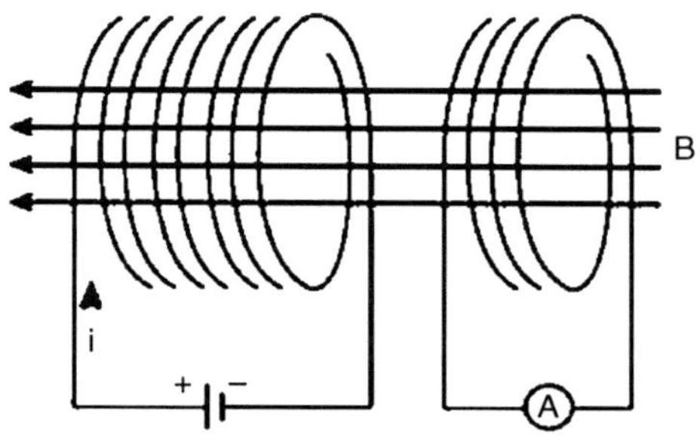

FIGURE 2.2 Mutual inductance.

The reluctance of a magnetic field R is similar to the resistance of an electric circuit and is the ratio of the magnetomotive force (mmf) to the total flux ϕ as expressed in Eq. (2.2):

$$R = \frac{\text{mmf}}{\phi} \tag{2.2}$$

The magnetomotive force (mmf) drives the flux ϕ in the circuit and is the total amount of electric current flowing in the coil, together with the total magnetic flux ϕ which is calculated from Eq. (2.3):

$$\phi = \int_A B dA \tag{2.3}$$

where B is the magnetic flux density, and A is cross-section area.

For a linear isotropic homogeneous magnetic material, the total reluctance is expressed as shown in Eq. (2.4):

$$R = \frac{l}{\mu A} \tag{2.4}$$

where l is length of the material, A is the uniform cross-sectional area and μ is the permeability of the material (H/m). Here μ is defined as μ_0 for a vacuum, air, or non-magnetic materials and its value is $4\pi \times 10^{-7}$ but, for magnetic materials, μ depends on both μ_0 and also μ_R which is the relative permeability of the material. Equation (2.4) indicates that the reluctance changes directly with length while it changes inversely with permeability of the material and the cross-sectional area.

Inductance or self-inductance L is defined by Eq. (2.5):

$$L = \frac{N\phi}{I} \tag{2.5}$$

where L is in henries, N is the number of turns in the coil, and ϕ is the flux of each turn of the coil. When the current changes in the circuit, a voltage V_L is induced in the circuit and is expressed as shown in Eq. (2.6):

$$V_L = \frac{Ldi}{dt} \tag{2.6}$$

When two coils are placed in close proximity to each other, as shown in Fig. 2.2, their magnetic fluxes affect each other to the extent that a change in current of one coil affects the magnetic flux, and therefore, the current, of the other coil. Hence, the inductance of each inductor changes and this property is known as mutual inductance.

2.2.1.3 Hall Effect and Magnetoresistance Effect

Hall effect and magnetoresistance effect are similar in that they both occur when a current-carrying conductor is subjected to a magnetic field. Devices utilizing both phenomena are used widely in industry. Hall-effect sensors are used as proximity sensors or proportional sensing devices. Hall-effect sensors are a very reliable, very cheap, and noncontact way of sensing magnetic objects. The magnetoresistance effect is used to measure the direct magnetic field, as well as those effects related to the measurement of other quantities by means of a magnetic field variation.

The Hall effect was first discovered in 1879 by Edwin Herbert Hall at Johns Hopkins University.[3] This effect is based on electrical conduction in a magnetic field. When a conductive material is subjected to a magnetic field, and an electric current flows perpendicular to the magnetic field, a voltage is generated in the conductor which is the Hall voltage V_H and its direction is perpendicular to both the magnetic field and the current, as shown in Fig. 2.3. The equation for the Hall voltage V_H is given in Eq. (2.7):[4]

$$V_H = \frac{R_H IB}{h} \tag{2.7}$$

where B is the magnetic field, I is the current, R_H is the Hall coefficient, and h is the width of the material (h is parallel with direction of B). The material used in the manufacture of Hall-effect devices is a p-type or an n-type semiconductor. R_H is negative for an n-type semiconductor.[4]

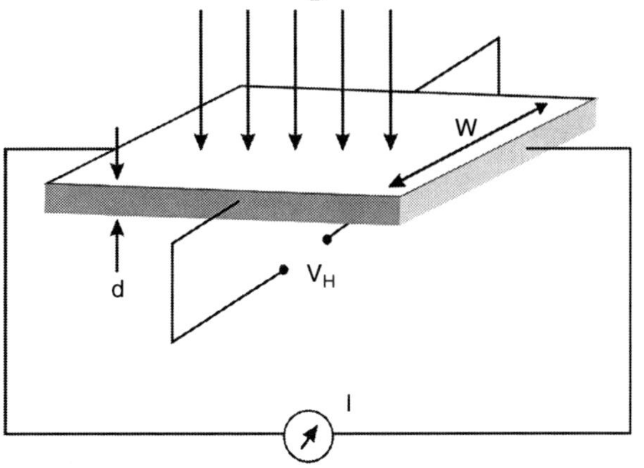

FIGURE 2.3 The Hall effect.

When a charged particle moves in a magnetic field, a laterally magnetic force perpendicular to both the magnetic field B and the velocity v of the charge q is applied on it. This force is known as the Lorentz force and is shown in Eq. (2.8):

$$\vec{F} = q\,\vec{v} \times \vec{B} \tag{2.8}$$

where $\vec{F}$ is the force, q is the electric charge of the particle, $\vec{v}$ is the velocity of the charged particle, and $\vec{B}$ is the magnetic field.

Magnetoresistance is the effect whereby the resistance of a conductor changes with the application of an external magnetic field and was discovered by Lord Kelvin in the 1850s. This discovery also showed that although both iron and nickel exhibit a small increase in electrical resistance along the direction of an applied magnetic field and a similar decrease occurred in resistance in the transverse direction, the magnitude of this effect depended on the material in question being greater in nickel than in iron.[6] Although Kelvin was unable to reduce the resistance in either material by more than 5 percent due to the fixed property inherent in each material, the pertinence of magnetoresistance (MR) has increased dramatically in this computer age because it is this very phenomenon that is used when reading bits on a disk. In order to store more bits on a disc, the bit has to, inevitably, become smaller and its magnetic field proportionately weaker. With the advent of new material and techniques, however, reductions in resistance of 50 percent or even greater is now possible which enables read/write heads to discern information in greatly reduced and weakened magnetic fields.

2.2.1.4 Resistance

Resistive transducers have various applications in mechatronics systems such as measuring displacement, force, pressure, mechanical strain, temperature, and fluid velocity.[4] The strength of the electric field in a bar of material is expressed as shown in Eq. (2.9):

$$E = \frac{V}{l} \tag{2.9}$$

where l is the length of the bar, V is the voltage of the battery connected to the ends of the bar and E is the electric field. The electric field causes free electrons to move in the opposite direction of the electric field and for electric current to flow through the material from the positive to negative ends of the battery. The electric current is the rate of electric charge flowing in the material and is calculated using Eq. (2.10):

$$I = \frac{dq}{dt} \tag{2.10}$$

where I is the electric current in amperes, q is the electric charge in coulombs, and t is the time in seconds. The electric current used in sensor technologies is usually much smaller than 1 A.[3]

The amount of electric current flowing in a material depends on the supply voltage V and its electrical resistance R, and it is defined by Eq. (2.11):

$$I = \frac{V}{R} \tag{2.11}$$

where R is the electrical resistance, V is the voltage, and I is the electric current. The change in any physical property that affects resistance characteristics can be measured by a resistive sensor.

2.2.1.5 Piezoelectricity

The piezoelectric effect is the property of crystalline materials used in piezoelectric sensors to measure pressure, acceleration, force, and strain. The piezoelectric effect exists in crystals such as quartz (SiO_2), tourmaline, and Rochelle salt. It also exists in polarized artificial ceramics, and polymers such as polyvinylidene fluoride (PVDF).[3,5] The word *piezo* is derived from the Greek word *piezein* meaning to press and the piezoelectric effect was first discovered in 1880 by the Curie brothers.

When piezoelectric material is subjected to mechanical stress or deformation, it generates an electrical voltage in proportion to the applied stress and, in like manner, it becomes mechanically deformed when it is subjected to an electric field.

At the molecular level, when neither stress nor deformation is applied on the piezoelectric material, its dipoles have random orientations in the structure of the material and there is no electric field. When the piezoelectric material is deformed or subjected to a mechanical stress, the dipoles become unbalanced and cause a net dipole moment that produces an electric field in the material. At normal temperatures, there is no center of symmetry in the crystalline structure of a ceramic. The crystalline structure of a ceramic is altered by increasing the temperature up to a certain value called the "Curie temperature" in which the dipole moment of the material is still zero as seen in Fig. 2.4. When the ceramic cools to below this temperature, the random structure of its dipoles returns to normal. By subjecting the material to an electric field while its temperature is cooling down, the dipoles will orientate in the direction of the applied force and the direction of the dipoles will remain unchanged even when the electrical field is removed. This process, leading to the formation of dipole moment within the bulk of the ceramic, is called poling.[7]

Piezoelectric ceramics and crystal materials are the two main groups of materials that are used in piezoelectric sensors. Piezoelectric ceramics have various advantages that make them more suitable than crystals to be used in piezoelectric sensors. Crystals are

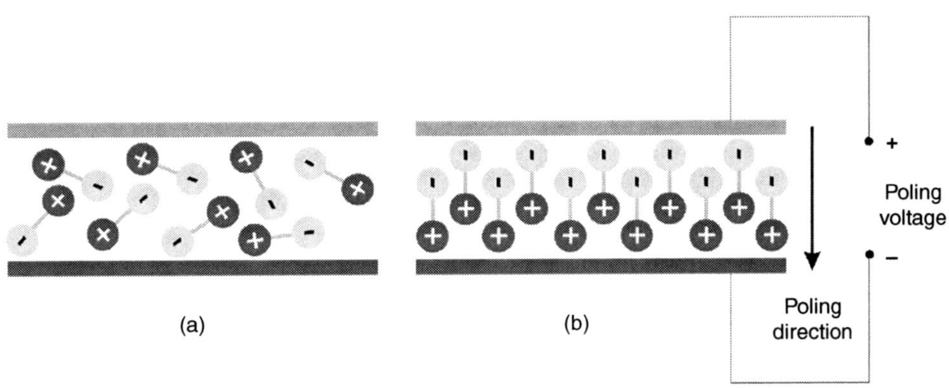

FIGURE 2.4 (*a*) Randomly directed dipoles in a piezoelectric material. (*b*) Alignment of dipoles in the direction of the electric field.

very rigid and large forces are required for generating an electric charge in crystals.[8] Some other advantages of ceramics are their high durability, high tensile strength, selective polarization direction, and construction in any size or shape.[5,7] Piezoelectric materials are also available in the form of films. Polyvinylidene fluoride (PVDF or PVF_2) is a piezoelectric polymeric film which is mechanically flexible and durable and can be fabricated in various shapes and can be as thin as 5 μm.[3,7] Piezoelectric films have low density, low acoustic impedance, excellent sensitivity, and 10 times greater compliance than that of ceramics.[3] By applying a compressive or tensile force on the PVDF film, a voltage is produced across the surface of the film that is proportional to the force applied.

A property of PVDF and other piezoelectric materials is the pyroelectric effect according to which an electrical charge is produced when the temperature of the material changes. Pyroelectric sensors act as a capacitor that can be charged electrically by a heat flow and, in this regard, operate more as heat-flow detectors rather than purely heat detectors.[3] The pyroelectric voltage output V in a film is calculated from Eq. (2.12):[7]

$$V = \frac{Ct\Delta T}{\varepsilon} \tag{2.12}$$

where C is the pyroelectric coefficient (C/m²·K), t is thickness of the film (m), T is the absolute temperature (K), and ε is the dielectric constant of the film (F/m).

Piezoelectric sensors are mainly used for measuring dynamic forces such as oscillation and impact. Because static loads result in a constant amount of charge on the piezoelectric material, these types of sensors are not, therefore, suitable for measuring static forces or pressures.

2.2.1.6 Light

Light is a form of electromagnetic radiation which has a wavelength in the range from about 0.1 to 100 μm.[3] Electromagnetic waves can travel through empty space without the need of any medium. The only electromagnetic waves that we are able to see are visible light waves. The shortest wavelength of visible light waves is violet; the longest wavelength is red. Beyond these wavelengths are infrared and ultraviolet.

Light can be used in optical sensors to detect physical properties such as distance, motion, shape, speed, and temperature. An optical sensor has a light emitter receiver and possesses the physical property to change the intensity of the light traveling from the emitter to the receiver.

The velocity of light in vacuum (c_0) is constant and independent of wavelengths as shown in Eq. (2.13):[3]

$$c_0 = \frac{1}{\sqrt{\mu_0 \varepsilon_0}} = 299{,}792{,}458.7 \pm 1.1 \ \frac{\text{m}}{\text{s}} \tag{2.13}$$

where $\mu_0 = 4\pi \times 10^{-7}$ H/m and $\varepsilon_0 = 8.854 \times 10^{-12}$ F/m are the magnetic and electric permitivities of free space.[3] The velocity of light can be applied to time-of-flight measurements to measure large distances with high precision.

The electric and magnetic fields are always perpendicular to each other for electromagnetic waves and are also perpendicular to the direction of propagation of the wave. As shown in Fig. 2.5, when the electromagnetic wave travels in the z direction, and the electric field oscillates in the xz plane, the magnetic field oscillates in the yz plane.

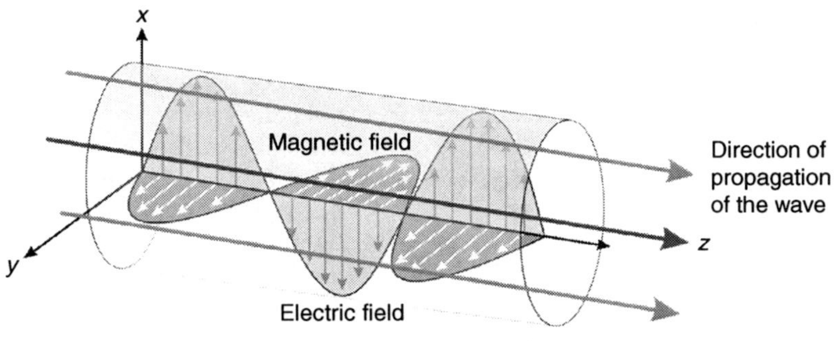

FIGURE 2.5 The electric and magnetic fields are always perpendicular to each other for electromagnetic waves and also perpendicular to the direction of propagation of the wave.

One of the properties of transverse waves, such as electromagnetic waves, is polarization, which means that all the electric field vectors are in one direction and parallel to each other. For example, when a polarized electromagnetic wave is propagating in the z direction, the electric field makes a unique angle with the x axis. But in a nonpolarized electromagnetic wave, the direction of the electric field is random and changes very quickly.

2.2.1.7 Sound Wave

Sound is a mechanical wave caused by the vibration of an object in a medium (solid, liquid, and gas). When the object vibrates, it sends a series of mechanical waves through the medium which are interpreted as sound. The range of audible sound for an average human ear is between 20 Hz and 20 kHz.[3] Sounds below this range (infrasound) and above this range (ultrasound) are usually inaudible. The speed of sound depends on the medium through which it is travelling and cannot travel through a vacuum at all. Sound waves are longitudinal and the vibration of particles is in the same direction as wave propagation.

Pressure applied on any medium causes its volume to change and the bulk modulus for an elastic medium is defined as the ratio of change in applied pressure ΔP to a relative change in the volume of the medium $(\Delta V/V)$. The bulk modulus of elasticity B can also be expressed as shown in Eq. (2.14):[3]

$$B = -\frac{\Delta P}{\Delta V/V} = \rho_0 v^2 \tag{2.14}$$

where ρ_0 is the density outside the compression area and v is the speed of sound in the medium. So, the speed of sound can be expressed as shown in Eq. (2.15):[3]

$$v = \sqrt{\frac{B}{\rho_0}} \tag{2.15}$$

From Eq. (2.15), it can be seen that the speed of sound in a medium is a function of the inertial property (density) and the elastic property (the bulk modulus of elasticity) of the medium and, since both of these properties depend on temperature, the speed of sound in a medium is a function of temperature.[3]

The intensity of a sound wave is the amount of power transmitted through a unit area. Sound is usually described by a parameter called the sound intensity level β which is defined as being the logarithmic ratio of the intensity of sound wave I to the reference sound intensity I_0. β is expressed as shown in Eq. (2. 16):

$$\beta = 10 \log_{10}\left(\frac{I}{I_0}\right) \tag{2.16}$$

where $I_0 = 10^{-12}$ (W/m^2) and the unit of β is decibel (dB).

2.2.2 Sensor Characterization

There are a number of different factors that should be taken into consideration when selecting the most suitable sensors for a mechatronics system, not the least of which is its purpose and application. Those most commonly used, together with their characterization, are explained in this section.

2.2.2.1 Transfer Function

Transfer function is the functional relationship between the physical input signal and the electrical output signal of a sensor.[9] The transfer function f, which can be either linear or nonlinear, represents the mathematical relationship between the input X and the output S and is expressed as $S = f(X)$. In many cases, the output is related to one input stimulus by the transfer function and the relationship is one dimensional as shown in Eq. (2.17):

$$S = a + bX \tag{2.17}$$

where a is the intercept (the output signal at zero input signal), b is the slope (sometimes called sensitivity), and S is one of the characteristics of the electrical output signal such as amplitude, frequency, or phase.[3]

In nonlinear transfer functions, b (the sensitivity) is not a fixed number and at any particular input value (X_0), b can be expressed as shown in Eq. (2.18):

$$b = \left.\frac{dS}{dX}\right|_{X=X_0} \tag{2.18}$$

The transfer function is the input-to-output relationship of a sensor, but for measuring a physical quantity by a sensor, its inversed transfer function (output-to-input) is required. Transfer functions are usually used in the analysis of systems in various fields, such as signal processing and control theory.

2.2.2.2 Accuracy

The *accuracy of a sensor* is defined as the largest deviation of a measured value from its true input value.[3] As an example, if we can consider a linear displacement sensor that has a linear transfer function with slope of b = 2 mV/mm, it follows that it ideally generates 2 mV per 1 mm displacement. In the experiment, an output of $S_{\text{exp.}} = 40.6$ mV is produced by a displacement of $X_{\text{true}} = 20$ mm. $X_{\text{exp.}}$ is calculated by using the inversed transfer function and is $X_{\text{exp.}} = S_{\text{exp.}}/b = 20.3$ mm. This means that the difference between the measured displacement in the experiment and the true displacement of the sensor is 0.3 mm which means that the sensor is accurate to within ±0.3 mm in a 20-mm range. When the experiment is repeated many times without any random error and the error is the same (±0.3 mm) in every repetition, it is said that the sensor has a systematic accuracy of ±0.3 mm over a 20-mm dynamic range of the sensor.[3]

2.2.2.3 Span

Span or input full scale (FS) is a dynamic range of stimuli which can be converted to electrical signals by a sensor without causing any unacceptably large inaccuracy.[3] *Span* can be also defined as the ratio of the maximum value of the physical input signal to the minimum value of the physical input signal that can be changed into electrical output signals by a sensor.[5] The dynamic range of the input physical signals is often represented in decibels for sensors with a very broad and nonlinear response characteristic. In these sensors, the dynamic range of the input physical signals is a logarithmic ratio of power or force. This ratio for power is expressed as shown in Eq. (2.19) and this ratio for force (current or voltage) is expressed as Eq. (2.20):[10]

$$1\ \text{dB} = 10 \times \log\frac{P_2}{P_1} \tag{2.19}$$

$$1\ \text{dB} = 20 \times \log\frac{X_2}{X_1} \tag{2.20}$$

Full-scale output (FSO) is defined as the algebraic difference between the electrical output signals measured with the maximum input stimulus and the minimum input stimulus applied on a sensor.[3]

2.2.2.4 Resolution

The resolution of a sensor is the smallest change it can detect in the quantity that it is measuring.[1] The resolution of the designed sensor should be lower than the smallest measurement which is required in the mechatronics system. For example, when the resolution of a distance-measuring sensor is 1 mm, the sensor can detect changes as small as 1 mm in distance. It means that when the change in distance is lower than 1 mm, the output signal of the sensor will not change.

The difference between accuracy and resolution is that accuracy is the closeness of a measurement to the actual value being measured whereas resolution is the smallest detectable increment to which an instrument can either measure or display.

2.2.2.5 Calibration

Calibration is the relationship between the input and output signal of a specific sensor.[11] To calibrate a sensor, a known physical input is applied to the system and the output signal is recorded and plotted on calibration curve. Linear calibration curves result in the best precision and accuracy and are more desirable. As shown in Fig. 2.6, the calibration curve is linear for input values less than X_l, and becomes nonlinear and less sensitive for input values greater than X_l. Nonlinearity of the calibration curve continues until it reaches a saturated value S_S of the output signal.[5] The inaccuracy allowed by a manufacturer when a sensor is calibrated in the factory is called the calibration error.[3]

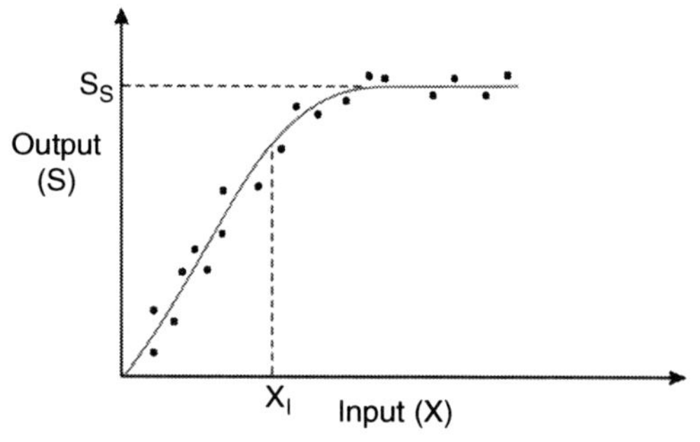

FIGURE 2.6 A typical calibration curve.

2.2.2.6 Nonlinearity

Nonlinearity is the maximum deviation of a real transfer function from the estimated straight line.[3] When the relationship between the input and output of a sensor follows a straight line, the sensor is seen to have a linear response. Linear systems can be calibrated more easily than nonlinear systems. There are several methods for superimposing a line on the transfer function and determining the nonlinearity. One method of superimposing a line on the transfer function is to use terminal points. In this method, a straight line is drawn through two points of output values at the maximum and minimum stimulus values.

2.2.2.7 Repeatability

Repeatability, or reproducibility, is the ability of a sensor to consistently show identical outputs for the same inputs. The repeatability error is the maximum difference between output values of two calibrating cycles and, because it represents the ability of the measurement process to repeat values in a short period of time, is the simplest measurement error to estimate.[3]

2.2.2.8 Reliability

Reliability is defined as the ability of a device (in this case a sensor) to perform a required function under stated conditions for a stated period of time otherwise known as the mean time between failures (MTBF).[3] There are two concepts for reliability; intrinsic reliability and achieved reliability.[12] Intrinsic reliability is the consistency in which a measurement technique can theoretically be successfully subjected to repeated trials whereas achieved reliability is its proven operational reliability.

2.2.2.9 Hysteresis

This is an error caused when the measured property reverses direction, but there is some finite lag in time for the sensor to respond, creating a different offset error in one direction than in the other. In some sensors, when the input stimulus of the sensor returns to its initial value in a path different from the one it had previously approached, the sensor does not reach the same output value. This is more comprehensible in cyclic inputs in which the input stimulus reaches the same value twice, both on its way and on its return. Regarding the output signal of a sensor, hysteresis is expressed as the difference between upscale and downscale approaches to the same position.[12] As shown in Fig. 2.7, in which this variation is shown graphically, the sensor has an increasing output as it crosses through position S. Then its direction is reversed and it has a decreasing output as it

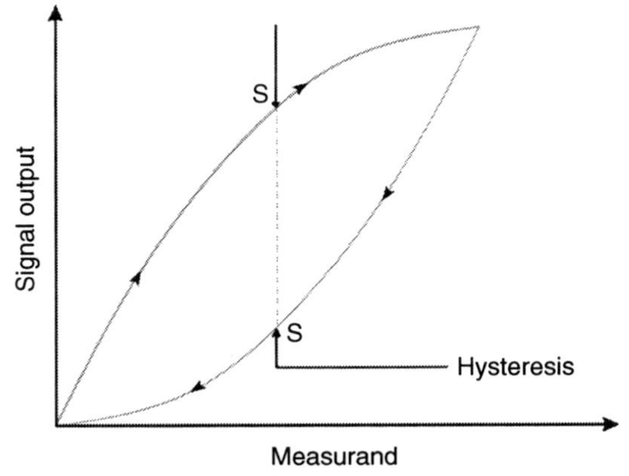

FIGURE 2.7 Hysteresis error in terms of the measured quantity.

passes again through position *S* toward zero. The variation in the reading recorded for the increasing and decreasing when it approaches position *S* is due to hysteresis that, in most types of material, mainly occurs due to inherent frictional and structural changes.[3]

2.2.2.10 Sensitivity

Sensitivity can be described as being the minimum input of a physical parameter that will create a detectable output change. In some sensors, the *sensitivity* is defined as the input parameter change required in order to produce a standardized output change.[9] Sensitivity of linear sensors is constant over the entire input range while sensitivity of nonlinear sensors increases or decreases as the input signal is changed.

2.2.2.11 Dead Band

Dead band is the insensitivity of a sensor in a specific range of input signals within which the output may remain at a certain value (often zero) over an entire dead band zone.[3] When the input signal transcends this band, the output varies with input. Figure 2.8 shows the dead band zone in a transfer function.

2.2.2.12 Response Time

The response time, shown as T_r in Fig. 2.9*a*, is the amount of time that lags between the application of an instantaneous change in the physical input to a sensor and the resulting indication of that change in the sensor output.[12] It is an indication of the fact that when the input signal changes in a sensor, the output signal does not change immediately. Another parameter relating to this concept is decay time which, as shown as T_d in Fig. 2.9*b*, is the time required in response to a negative going step-function change of the input parameter.[13] In Fig. 2.9, T_{on} is the onset time of the input signal and T_{off} is the offset time of the input signal.

2.2.2.13 Noise

Noise is the undesirable signals that arise in the sensor output and not caused by the sensor input.[14] There are two basic classifications of inherent noise for any given circuit, namely interference noise and transmitted noise.[3] Interference noise is that which arises within the circuit itself whereas interference noise is that which is picked up from outside

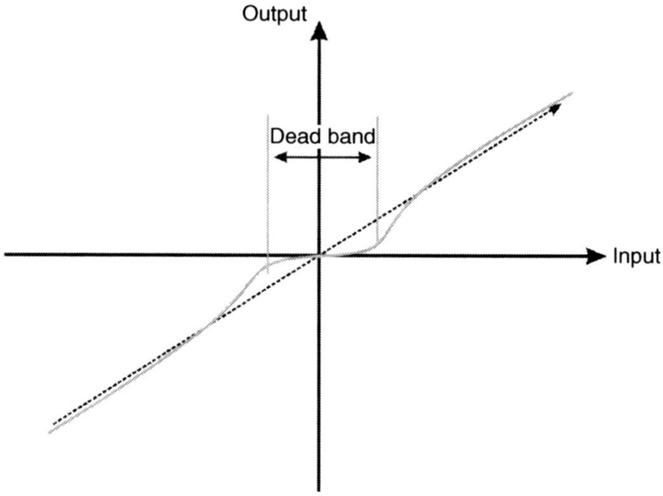

FIGURE 2.8 The dead band zone.

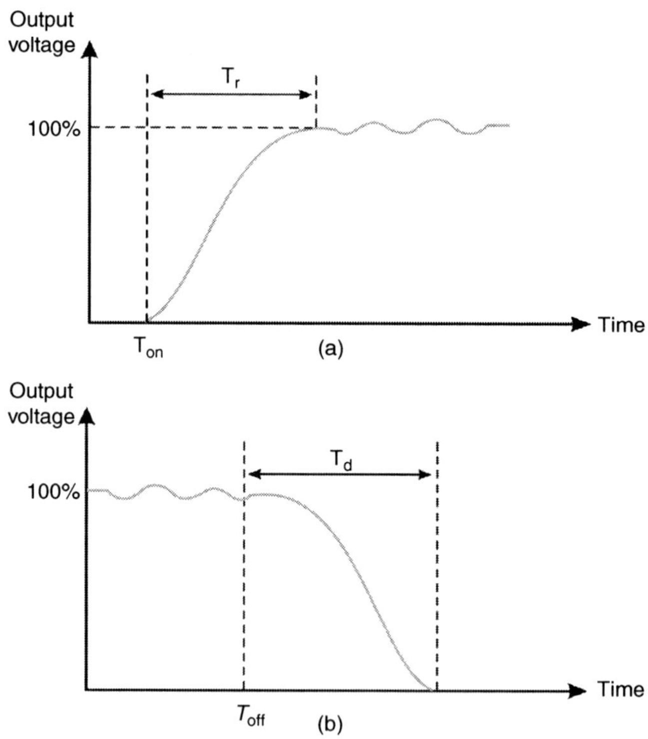

FIGURE 2.9 (*a*) Response time. (*b*) Decay time.

the circuit. In general, because noise may cause considerable errors in the system, sensors that are immune to noise should be employed whenever this factor is an issue. These include capacitor, piezoelectric, ultrasonic, and focused-laser (FL) interferometric. These are ideal, provided that they also fulfill the criteria of size, weight, and cost.

2.2.3 Sensors

Many different types of sensors can be used for any desired physical phenomenon and application; in this section, the most common ones are discussed. The classification of sensors is usually formulated by their application in detecting and measuring physical quantities such as displacement, force, pressure, velocity, acceleration, temperature, strain, and flow by converting these phenomena into electrical signals.

2.2.3.1 Position and Displacement Sensors

Position is expressed as the determination of an object's coordinates with regard to a selected reference point and displacement is expressed as the object moving from one position to another by a specific distance or angle.[3] Position and displacement measurements have many applications, such as those that are used in robotics, performance evaluation, process feedback control, and security systems. Here, some of the most common position and displacement sensors are explained.

Linear Variable Differential Transformer The linear variable differential transformer (LVDT) is an electromechanical displacement sensor consisting of a primary coil, two adjacent secondary coils, and a ferromagnetic core that can move axially within the coils. A typical structure of an LVDT is shown in Fig. 2.10. As shown in this figure, two secondary

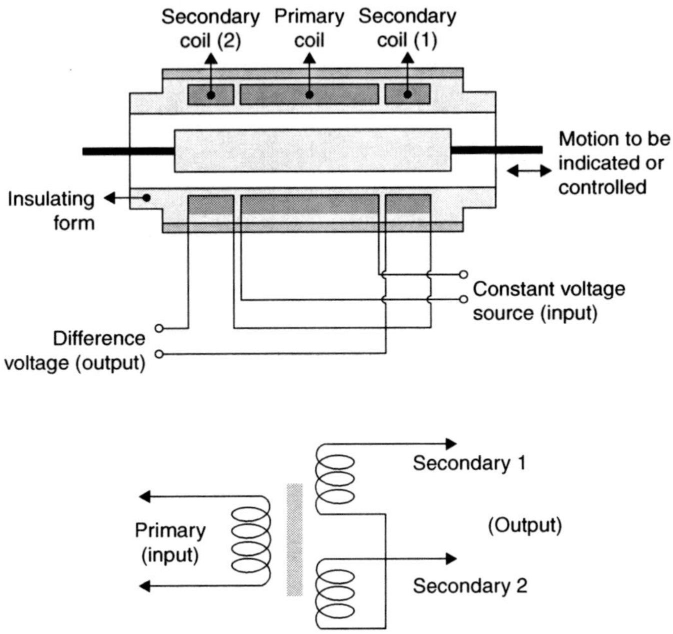

FIGURE 2.10 A typical structure of an LVDT. (From Najarian et al., Artificial Tactile Sensing in Biomedical Engineering, McGraw-Hill, USA, 2009. Reproduced with permission of The McGraw-Hill Companies, Inc.)

coils are symmetrically placed around the primary coil. The core is in contact with the target object in motion. An external AC power source energizes the primary coil and, because of coupling of magnetic flux between the coils, AC voltages are induced in the secondary coils. When the core is located in the magnetic center of the LVDT, the secondary output signals cancel each other out and there is no output voltage. As the core moves in the LVDT coil, the reluctance of the flux path changes. The magnitude of the output signal of the LVDT is proportional to the position of the core within the magnetic center of the LVDT.

Over a large range of core displacement, the LVDT can operate linearly. When the core passes the center position, the phase changes by 180 degrees and this phase change shows the direction in which the core is moving. This moving pattern and phase change is illustrated in Fig. 2.11.

Rotary Variable Differential Transformer The rotary variable differential transformer (RVDT) is an angular displacement sensor which operates in a similar manner to the LVDT, the only difference being that it has a rotary ferromagnetic core.

Incremental Encoders Incremental encoders are position feedback devices. Linear encoders measure linear position and direction, and rotary encoders measure the angular position and direction of a motor or mechanical drive shaft. In a rotary incremental encoder, a glass or metal disk with a pattern of opaque and transparent sectors is attached to a shaft. The pattern is a code track. A light source and a photodetector are placed on opposite sides of the disk (Fig. 2.12). As the disk rotates with the motor shaft, the code track interrupts the light emitted onto the photodetector and a digital signal output is produced.

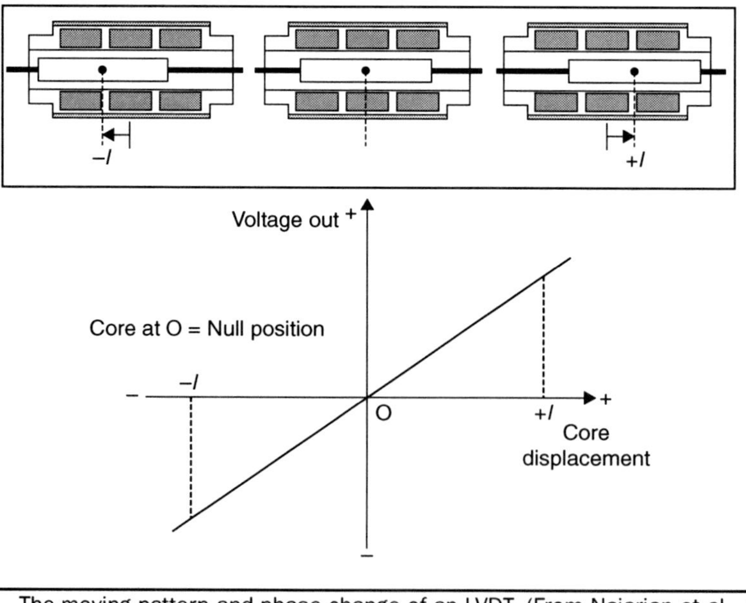

FIGURE 2.11 The moving pattern and phase change of an LVDT. (From Najarian et al., Artificial Tactile Sensing in Biomedical Engineering, McGraw-Hill, USA, 2009. Reproduced with permission of The McGraw-Hill Companies, Inc.)

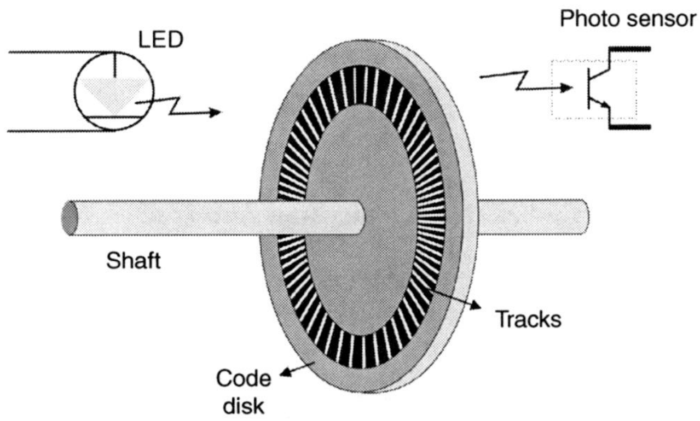

FIGURE 2.12 The rotary optical encoder.

The number of cycles the encoder will output per revolution corresponds to the number of opaque and transparent sector pairs on the code track. The base resolution of the encoder is determined by the number of cycles per revolution (CPR).[15] In incremental encoders, the feedback signal is referenced to a start or home position and provides relative position.

Absolute Encoders An absolute encoder, shown in Fig. 2.13, is similar to an incremental encoder, the only difference being that the disk attached on the motor or mechanical drive shaft has multiple concentric code tracks for each of which a separate photo detector is used. The binary resolution of the encoder is equivalent to the number of code tracks and among the most commonly used are binary encoders having resolutions of 8, 10, and 12 bits. Since absolute encoders have various output formats, the compatibility of the robot controller or intelligent drive with the particular model of the absolute encoder should be ensured.[15]

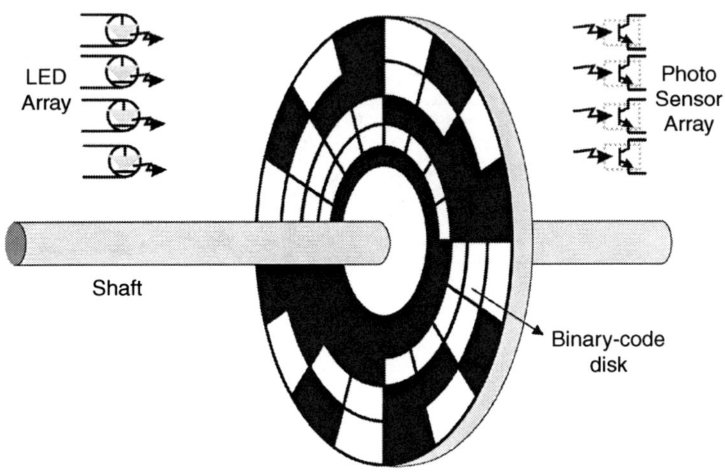

FIGURE 2.13 Absolute optical rotary encoder.

An important feature of an absolute encoder is that its code track keeps the last angular position of the encoder shaft whenever it stops moving, whether the system is shut down intentionally or as a result of power failure. Hence, an absolute encoder is used in systems in which the position of the motors is needed immediately upon system start-up.

Resolver A resolver is basically a rotary transformer that can provide absolute position information over one revolution.[15] Resolvers, which can be an alternative to encoders for joint feedback in robotic applications, consist of a primary coil placed on the rotor and a pair of secondary coils placed on the stator. The secondary coils are oriented 90 degrees relative to each other. A schematic of a resolver is shown in Fig. 2.14.

When an AC reference signal is applied to the rotor coil, it produces an AC voltage output that changes in amplitude according to the sine and cosine of the shaft position. The phase shift angle between the applied signal to the rotor and the induced signal appearing on the stator coil is an analog representation of the rotor position.[16] When the resolver shaft turns through one revolution, the absolute position of the load being driven is the ratio of the sine output amplitude to the cosine output amplitude.

Potentiometer Potentiometers are variable resistance devices applicable in contact displacement measurement. A change in the linear or angular displacement of a potentiometer changes the effective length of its conductor, and so, the resistance of the device. A movable slide or wiper attached to the target object in motion is in contact with a resistive material or wire coil. A potentiometer is shown in Fig. 2.15. A voltage is applied to the resistive material and when the slide moves relative to the material, the output voltage changes linearly with the total resistance. Potentiometers have a tendency for nonlinearity and they should be used carefully when a high degree of accuracy is required.[17]

Laser Inferometer Laser interferometers give the most accurate position feedback for servosystems.[16] In laser interferometers, the laser source sends the light to a polarizing

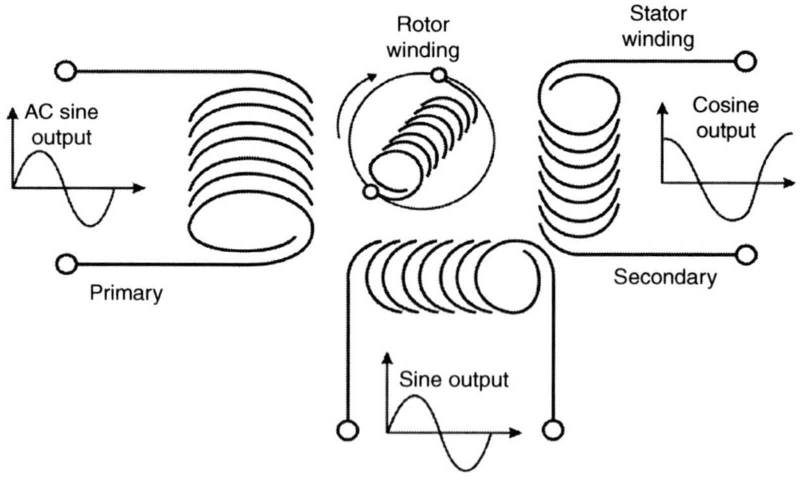

Figure 2.14 Schematic of a resolver.

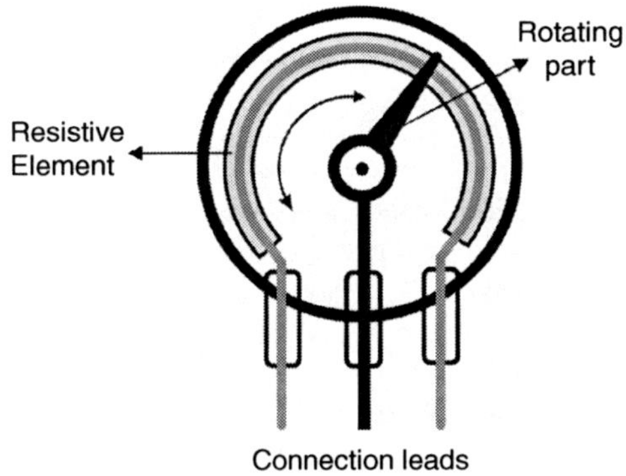

Figure 2.15 Schematic of a potentiometer.

beam splitter which divides the light into two parts, one of which goes straight through the polarizing beam splitter and the other is reflected. The part that goes straight through the beam splitter reaches the moving reflectometer and is reflected back to the beam splitter that passes it on to the photodetector. The part of the beam that is reflected by the beam splitter reaches the fixed retroreflector placed at a certain distance. The retroreflector reflects the beam back to the beam splitter before it is reflected into the photodetector. So, the two reflected laser beams strike the photodetector, and the combination of the two light beams is changed into an electrical signal. A diagram of a laser interferometer is shown in Fig. 2.16. The position measurement in laser interferometers depends only on the difference in distance between the round trip laser beam travels from the beam splitter to the moving retroreflector and the fixed round trip distance of laser beam travel from the beam splitter to the fixed retroreflector.[16]

Proximity Sensors Proximity sensors are used for detecting the presence of an object. A proximity sensor is a threshold version of a position sensor and generates the output signal when a certain distance to the object becomes necessary for an indication.[3] Proximity sensors can be categorized into inductive, capacitive, and photoelectric sensors.[17]

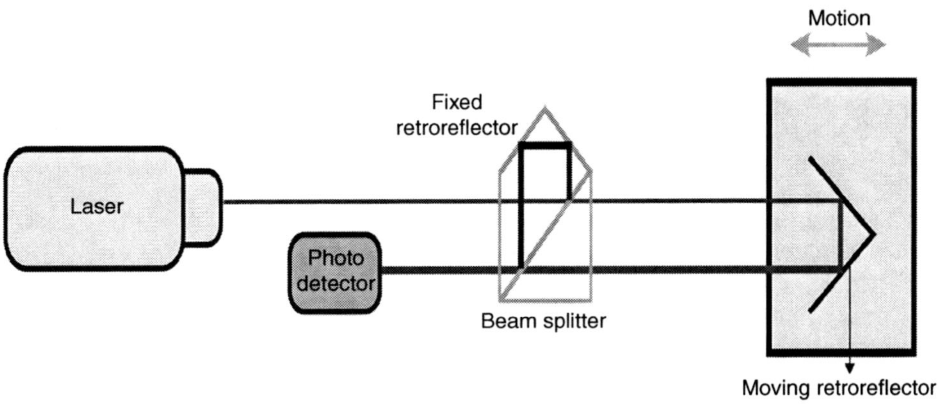

Figure 2.16 Diagram of a laser interferometer.

Inductive proximity sensors only detect the presence of ferrous and nonferrous metals but capacitance proximity sensors detect the presence of almost any material. Photoelectric proximity sensors have various configurations and include an infrared light-emitting diode (LED) source and a light sensitive switch as a detector.

2.2.3.2 Velocity and Acceleration Sensors

The measurement of velocity is applicable in the control of mechanical systems motion and measurement of acceleration is applicable in any system that is subject to shock and vibration. Although velocity and acceleration can be derived from the time history data achieved from linear or rotary sensors, velocity and acceleration sensors (whose output is directly proportional to velocity and acceleration) are preferred. Some of the most common velocity and acceleration sensors are discussed below.

Tachometer The tachometer is an incremental encoder with a single photodetector that provides velocity feedback for servosystems.[7] The frequency of the tachometer's output pulses signifies the rotational speed of the shaft. For controlling the drive motor and load speed, a tachometer is mechanically coupled to the DC motor and sends feedback signals to the controller and amplifier.

Accelerometer Accelerometers are used to measure acceleration. Two common types of accelerometers are the seismic mass type accelerometers and piezoelectric accelerometers. The principle of operation for a seismic mass type accelerometer is its relative motion between a mass and the supporting structure and is suitable for low to medium frequency applications. Piezoelectric accelerometers are compact and more suitable for high-frequency applications.[1]

2.2.3.3 Strain, Force, Pressure, and Tactile Sensors

Strain is defined as the amount of deformation per unit length of an object when an external force is applied. The most common strain sensor used in mechatronics is the strain gauge. The strain gauge is the basic element for various types of sensors such as force sensors, pressure sensors, and tactile sensors. Tactile sensors are a special type of force or pressure sensors. Here, strain gauges, tactile sensors, force sensors, and pressure sensors are described.

Strain Gauges A strain gauge is a resistive elastic sensor in which its electrical resistance changes as a function of the input strain which may be either positive (tensile) or negative (compressive). Because most materials tend to resist deformation, an applied force is necessary to cause deformation. So, resistance can be related to applied force. A bonded metallic strain gauge is composed of an insulating carrier, a foil or wire grid bonded to the insulating carrier, and an additional insulating layer attached to the top of the grid. The grid legs of the sensor are aligned with the required direction of strain measurement. A bonded metallic strain gauge is shown in Fig. 2.17. The grid is most sensitive to strain along its length. The gauge factor of the strain gauge is determined by the manufacturer.

Because resistance is a function of temperature, strain gauges are also sensitive to variations in temperature for which there must be compensation in order to obtain an accurate force measurement.

In order to measure strain with a bonded resistance strain gauge, it must be connected to a Wheatstone bridge circuit to measure the minute changes in resistance corresponding

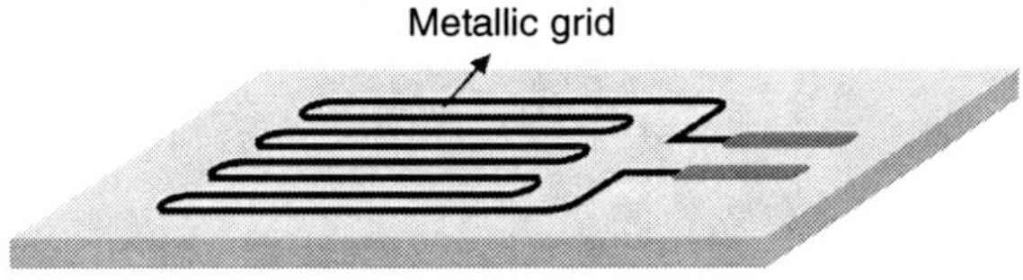

FIGURE 2.17 A schematic of a strain gauge sensor.

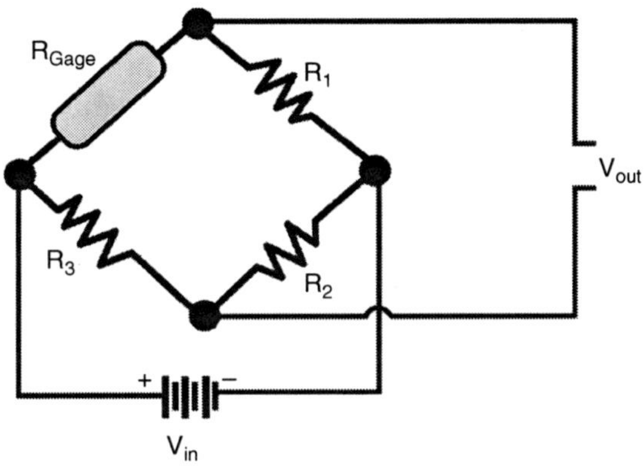

FIGURE 2.18 Typical Wheatstone bridge.

to strain. A typical Wheatstone bridge circuit is shown in Fig. 2.18. When force is applied to the bonded strain gauge, resistive changes take place and unbalance the Wheatstone bridge. The Wheatstone circuit is also used for temperature compensation.

Force Sensors Force sensors are useful in controlling mechanical systems. They also have many applications in robotic surgery including manipulation of soft tissue, suturing, tissue cutting, tissue recognition, needle insertion, and detection of an embedded object in tissue. Some types of force sensors are based on the technique of measuring a deflection caused by an applied force. In this technique, relatively high deflections (about several micrometers) are necessary to be feasible.[1] One example of these types of force sensor is helical springs that have excellent elastic properties and can transform the load to be measured into a deflection.

A common type of force sensor is the load cell which is available in various designs. One of the most popular types of load cells is the strain gauge load cell which is relatively accurate and is used for sensing large, static, or slowly varying forces with little deflection.[1] A typical load cell is shown in Fig. 2.19.

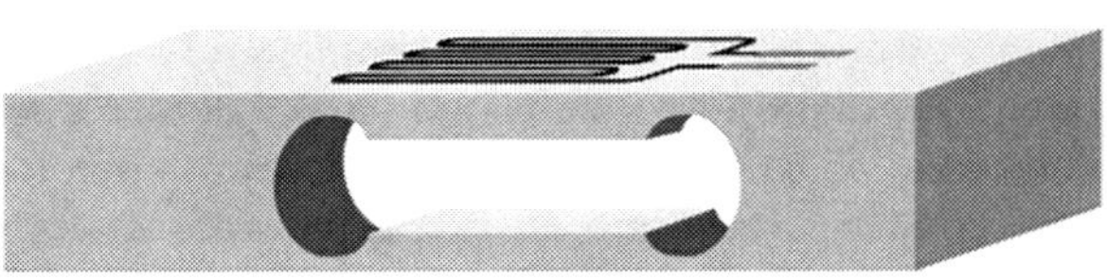

FIGURE 2.19 Schematic of a load cell.

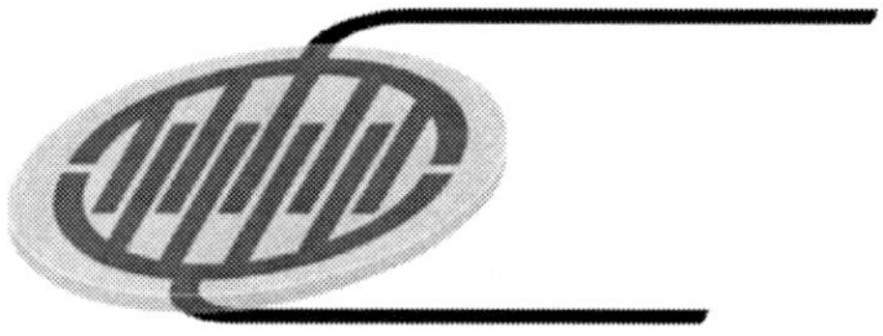

FIGURE 2.20 A schematic of a force sensing resistor (FSR).

Another type of force sensor is the piezoelectric force sensor in which, when a mechanical load is applied on its piezoelectric material, an electrostatic charge is developed in the material. This electrostatic charge is collected by electrodes and changed to an output voltage signal by using a charge amplifier. Piezoelectric sensors are used for dynamic measurements although, because of the leakage across their electrodes, they cannot measure static deflection.[15]

Force sensing resistors (FSRs) are another type of force sensors that are based on the technique of decreasing the resistance of polymer thick-film devices with the increase of an applied force. A force sensing resistor, shown in Fig. 2.20, is composed of a resistive material applied to a film and a set of digital-type contacts applied to another film. The resistive material is used for completing the electrical circuit between the two sets of conductors on the other film. When a force is applied to the FSR, a better connection is made between the contacts resulting in increased conductivity. FSRs are not suitable for accurate measurements of force because sensor parts display a 15 to 25 percent variation in resistance between each other.[1]

Pressure Sensors Pressure sensors have many applications in industrial and medical control and monitoring procedures. Some applications of pressure sensors in medicine and health monitoring are blood pressure measurement, abdominal pressure measurement, and foot pressure. *Pressure* is defined as force applied over an area and a force sensor can measure pressure when the area can be defined and held constant. Pressure sensors usually use a secondary force or displacement sensor to measure elastic deformation or displacement of a mechanical element such as a diaphragm, bellows, or optical fiber. Micropressure sensors consist of diaphragms that deform as a result of pressure differences. The diaphragm is an important element in most pressure sensors because it is the displacement of the diaghram that is measured by using capacitive sensing or piezoresistive sensing.

The time-of-flight sensor is another type of pressure sensor which can measure displacement caused by an applied pressure. They work by measuring the distance of an object by sending a signal or pulse of energy and measuring the time it takes for the reflected wave to return.[18]

Tactile Sensors Tactile sensation is the process of determining physical properties and events of an object through actual physical contact and a tactile sensing system detects and collects such information by means of an array of tactile sensors. A *tactile sensor* is defined as a sensor capable of detecting and measuring a given property of an object by making physical contact with it and changing that information into a form which can be processed. This means that tactile sensing is the process of detecting and measuring the spatial distribution of forces on a sensory area.[5]

Tactile sensing plays an important role in grasping and object identification. Tactile sensors have many applications in industry and clinical applications. In robotics, tactile sensors can be located on the fingertips of a mechanical actuator in order to provide information about the contact object. A robot acts as an information-processing system when a tactile sensor is mounted on its gripper and, based on information received from the tactile sensor, the motion of the robot could be controlled by the system.[14]

In a tactile sensing system, a closely spaced array of force sensors can be used to measure the force distribution and includes a regular pattern of sensing elements. Signals of a tactile array sensor provide dynamic contact information such as contact location, object shape, and the pressure distribution, but a strain gauge force sensor provides static grasp force information.[1]

2.2.3.4 Flow Sensors

Flow sensors are used for measuring the flow rate of a fluid. There are various types of flow sensors. The orifice plate and venture meter restrict the flow and determine the flow rate according to the pressure difference. The pitot tube is a pressure measurement instrument positioned against the flow and is used to measure the flow velocity and in turn the flow rate. The rotameter is a device that is located in the flow path and rotates at a speed proportional to the flow rate. In the following section, thermal transport flow sensors and ultrasonic flow sensors as two common flow sensors are explained.

Thermal Transport Flow Sensor Flow rate of a medium can be measured by marking the medium and then detecting the movement of the mark. The mark can be an object moving with the medium or stationary with respect to it. The flow rate is calculated according to the time that the object moves from one position in the flow to another position. Such an object may be a float, radioactive element, dye, and a different gas or liquid whose concentration and rate of dilution can be detected by proper sensors.[3] Instead of using an object as a mark, some physical properties of the moving medium such as its temperature can be changed. Then the rate of displacement of the changed medium or rate of its dilution can be measured.

In flow sensors based on thermal transport principles, a heated element is used that has a temperature slightly greater than the temperature of the ambient fluid.[1] The heat is generally generated by passing current through a resistive element. The movement of the fluid generates velocity-dependent forced convection of heat and, so, decreases the temperature of the heated element. Some information about the flow rate can be provided by the temperature of the element.

Ultrasonic Flow Sensor Ultrasonic flow sensors are used to measure flow rate without a direct contact with the fluid. These sensors measure fluid velocity by sending high-frequency sound waves through the fluid. The effective velocity of sound in a flowing medium is a sum of the velocity of sound relative to the medium and the velocity of the medium with respect to the source of the sound. Hence, sound waves spreading upstream will have a smaller effective velocity, and sound waves spreading downstream will have a higher effective velocity. Since the difference between the velocities in upstream and downstream is twice the velocity of the medium, the velocity of the flow can be determined by measuring the difference between the upstream/downstream velocities.[3]

2.2.3.5 Temperature Sensors

A temperature sensor converts thermal energy into an electrical signal and can operate in either contact or noncontact systems. In contact temperature sensors, heat conduction takes place through the interface between the object and the sensor in which part of the body's thermal radiation is absorbed by the contact temperature sensor and changed into a useful signal. In noncontact temperature sensors, there is no heat absorption from the body or tissue being monitored, and the advantage of these sensors is that temperature can be measured from a distance. Noncontact temperature sensors based on the principles of radiation thermometry have been developed recently for medical use.[17]

All temperature sensors can be divided into two categories, namely, absolute sensors and relative sensors.[3] An absolute temperature sensor measures the temperature with reference to either absolute zero or any other point on a temperature scale. A relative sensor measures the temperature difference between two objects while one object is the reference. As an example, thermistors and resistance temperature detectors (RTDs) are absolute sensors and thermocouples are relative sensors. These sensors are explained below.

Thermistors Thermistors are temperature sensitive resistors that can be classified into those having a positive temperature coefficient (PTC) and those with a negative temperature coefficient (NTC). PTC thermistors are made from barium and strontium titanate mixtures, while NTC thermistors are generally made from metallic oxides.[17] Thermistors operate as absolute temperature sensors and their characteristics are based on zero-power resistance.[3] This means that when an electric current passes through a thermistor, it does not cause any temperature increase (self heating) in the thermistor and so, it does not have any effect on the accuracy of measurement.

Resistance Temperature Detectors Resistance temperature detectors (RTDs) are generally metal sensors that are fabricated in the form of wires or thin films. The principle of operation of RTDs is changing the resistance of the metals with temperature. All RTDs have PTCs. Platinum, nickel, and copper wires are used in RTDs. Sources of error in RTD devices include their poor wire contact, thermoelectric electromotive forces, and self heating of the wire from passing current flow through the wire.[17]

Thermocouples A practical thermocouple consists of two wires of dissimilar metals that are electrically joined at one end (the measuring junction), and thermally joined at the other end (the reference junction). A low DC voltage is produced by the thermocouple when the two junctions are at different temperatures. This voltage is referred to as the thermoelectric voltage and is produced by the temperature gradient along the thermocouple wires. A typical thermocouple is shown in Fig. 2.21.

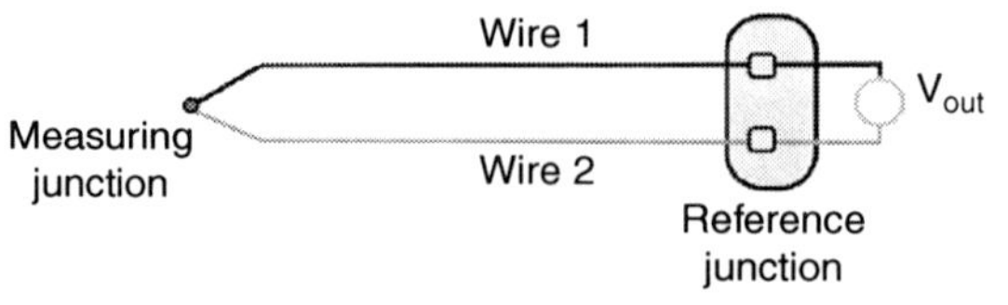

FIGURE 2.21 Schematic presentation of a typical thermocouple.

2.2.3.6 Chemical Sensors

A chemical sensor is a small device that, as the result of a chemical interaction or process between an analyte gas and the sensor device, transforms chemical or biochemical information of a quantitative or qualitative type into an analytically useful signal. These sensors are concerned with measuring chemical quantities such as identifying the presence of particular chemical compounds, detecting the concentration of various chemical species, and monitoring chemical activities in the body for diagnostic and therapeutic applications.[3] Chemical sensors have many applications in medicine. For example, these sensors can be used in monitoring oxygen in the lungs and in blood samples to give information about patient health. Here, some of the most common chemical sensors are explained.

ChemFET A ChemFET is a chemical field-effect transistor that contains a gas-selective coating or series of coatings between the transistor gate and the analyte.[3] In fact, chemFET is a chemically controlled resistor that is used to detect atoms, molecules, and ions in liquids and gases. ChemFETs are applicable in detecting O_2 in blood, H_2 in air, military nerve gases, NH_3, CO_2, and explosive gases.[19] The chemical-selective gate material of the chemFET changes the potential at which the device begins to conduct and thus indicates the presence of specific chemical species. A subtype of chemFET devices is ion-sensitive field-effect transistors (ISFET) which are used to detect ions in electrolytes. Another subtype of chemFET devices is enzyme field-effect transistors (ENFET) which are specialized for detection of specific enzymes and can operate as biochemical sensors.

Biochemical Sensors A biochemical sensor is a chemical sensor used in medical diagnosis and monitoring patient health. Biosensors sensors convert a biological response into an electrical signal. Biological elements such as organisms, tissues, cells, organelles, membranes, enzymes, receptors, antibodies, and nucleic acids may be detected qualitatively and quantitatively using biosensors.[20] An important issue in the fabrication of biosensors is immobilization of analytes on the physical sensor. Biosensors for *in vivo* and *in vitro* clinical analysis need special requirements. These include sterilization protocols to avoid denaturation of immobilized biological element and the necessary diffusion of the analyte from undiluted sample into the active bioselective layer. In addition, clinical biosensors require periodical recalibration and to invoke means by which it will never leak.[3]

The sensors discussed above are by no means exhaustive but are among the most common and applicable sensors used in mechatronics systems. A number of specialized sensors applicable in medicine are discussed in Sec. 2.4.

2.3 Machine Vision

Of the five senses with which we are conferred, vision is generally considered to be the most valuable. It provides most of the data that we receive and allows us to get information from the environment in order to guide our decisions and actions. Human image analysis is a multilayered process. It begins with simple graphical processing that is performed without our conscious awareness. Changes are brought to our attention. Then the images are coded in terms of lines, the curves and boundaries between two regions and, finally, we understand the shape. This type of perception is exemplified by the technology pioneered by Alta Vista in 1997, in which web services were protected by security protocols that were able to differentiate between a human user and a machine user.

The mechanism governing human vision is briefly described as follows:

1. The eye lens focuses rays of light emitted by objects in the outside world onto the retina. The lens is a transparent structure in the eye which changes the focal distance of the eye and allows a person to focus on objects at various distances. This adjustment of the eyes is controlled by the nervous system and is executed by the ciliary muscles around the lens.
2. The retina is a light-sensitive membrane in the back of the eye. It contains millions of photoreceptor cells and serves as a transducer for changing patterns of light into neuronal signals. These cells detect the photons of light and respond by generating neural impulses.
3. A network of neurons collects these impulses and transmits them down the optic nerve to the primary and secondary visual cortex of the brain. The brain then interprets these impulses into vision and constructs the image.
4. The visual information from each eye is carried to the primary visual cortex separately. By receiving separate information at the same time from both eyes, the primary visual cortex can figure the three-dimensional aspect. The primary visual cortex separates the image into distinct feature channels and the information is sent to the other visual-related areas of the brain. Different groups of cells work together to extract features such as color, depth, and edges.

The addition of vision to machines is a very great improvement and plays an important role in creating a model of the real world from images, and analysis and information management of the collected data. For example, it helps a physician to recover information by enhancing images and can be useful in different aspects of health care. Similar applications of the addition of vision to machines are inspection of industrial, agricultural, and a host of other fields.

Machine vision systems are devices that capture and analyze visual information, and are used to automate tasks that require visual perception. As such, they employ integrated mechanical-electronic-software systems for examining natural and man-made objects and materials, as well as manufacturing processes, in order to detect defects and improve quality, operating efficiency, the safety of products and processes, and control machines used in manufacturing.[21]

A typical machine vision system consists of most of the following components:

- An adequate light source together with one or more cameras capable of displaying the desired field of view onto the image sensor.
- Input/output hardware or communication links to report findings and results.
- A synchronizing sensor for part detection to trigger image acquisition and processing.
- A program to process images and detect related features.

Machine vision integrates image capture systems with digital input/output devices and computer networks to control manufacturing equipment such as robotic arms (Fig. 2.22).

Machine vision is actually concerned with a very diverse range of technologies and applications and is applied for visual inspections that require high-speed, high-magnification, 24-hour operation, and/or repeatability of measurements.

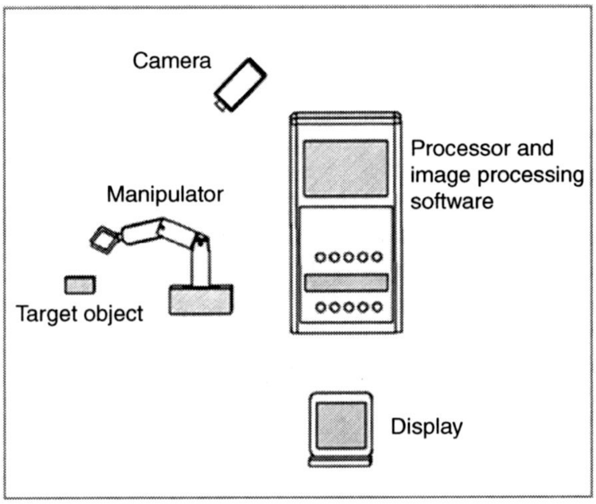

FIGURE 2.22 Diagram of a machine vision system.

Machine vision algorithms take images as inputs and generate other types of outputs, such as representations for the object contours in an image. Displaying images can also be used in machine vision applications and display functions are used for visualizing image data, recovering generated events and the associated data from an image display environment, selecting regions of interest from an image interactively, and annotating the image with additional information.[22]

All mechanical, optical, and electronic components, which are required to produce an image, can be described as a camera or camera system. A sensor is required in the camera to act as its eye. The camera's sensor is applied for capturing the image and translating it into information, which can either be preprocessed in the camera, or transmitted to a host or a monitor, and processed. To interpret and determine colors, the information of three (or four) pixels with different color perceptions should be combined. Red, green, and blue (RGB) or the complementary colors cyan, yellow, and magenta are typical triples to determine the color values.

The heart of a machine vision system is image processing which refers to the creation, acquisition, and analysis of images.[22] Image processing algorithms are used to enhance particular information and suppress noise.[23]

Computer graphics produce images from basic geometric shapes such as lines, circles, and free-form surfaces, but machine vision is an inverse problem and estimates the basic geometric shapes and other features from the image. Machine vision uses curve and surface representations and several other techniques from computer graphics which, in turn, utilize various techniques from machine vision to enter models into the computer for creating real images.

Pattern recognition is necessary for recognizing objects. *Object recognition* is defined as identification of objects using characteristic features such as geometry, dimensions, color, structure, and texture. Object identification includes the distinction of object variants and has many applications. For example, prior identification of correct objects in any given situation is required for position recognition or completeness checks.

2.4 Sensors Applications in Medicine

Sensors have many applications in medicine and can be integrated into devices used in surgical procedures as well as equipment used in intensive care units (ICUs), hospital recuperative care, and home care. Sensors can be miniaturized such that they can even measure different parameters at the place of origin in an invasive manner. One of the most useful applications of sensors in medicine is distance monitoring of vital medical parameters such as blood pressure, blood oxygen (SpO_2), pulse rate, respiration rate, blood glucose, etc. Such sensors provide real-time medical data transfer and communication without human control which therefore place them in high demand.

In the following section, various types of sensors are discussed including implantable sensors, temporarily inserted sensors, external sensors exposed to body fluids, and sensors used for external applications.

2.4.1 Implantable Sensors

Implantable sensors measure parameters inside the body and are used for detecting and monitoring medical conditions such as diabetes and heart disease. These types of sensors must, by necessity, be small, reliable, and biocompatible. They must also consume very little power and be long-lasting.

Piezoelectric polymer sensors are an example of implantable sensors which can be used in pacemakers to monitor activities of the patient and, furthermore, require no power.[24] This type of sensor employs a very small cantilever beam in which a weight attached on its end flops with patient body movements and transmits signals accordingly. Since the output of this sensor is incumbent upon bodily movement, the pacemaker is therefore able to ensure, in a commensurate manner, that the heartbeat is in accordance with these output signals. Figure 2.23 shows a pacemaker containing a miniature piezo film vibration sensor.

Implanted sensors can, however, also be charged from external sources. For instance, when a radio frequency (RF) energy wand is placed in close proximity to a sensor implanted inside the body that is alert to the advent of RF transmission, the sensor activates, measures the required parameter, sends the data back to the wand by RF link, and then deactivates.[24]

2.4.2 Temporary Inserted Sensors

Sometimes sensors are inserted into the body for either a matter of minutes or hours and can work with or without an external power source.

Catheter ablation sensors are an example of sensors that are inserted temporarily.[24] Catheter ablation is an invasive procedure, in which RF energy is often used to remove a faulty electrical pathway from the heart to correct abnormal arrhythmias. The force applied by the catheter tip to the target tissue must be less than predetermined values in order to prevent the tissue from perforating. A triaxial force-sensing system can be used to measure contact forces of tissue in all three dimensions simultaneously.

Fetal monitoring is an electronic method to record the vital physiologic functions during pregnancy and birth. This technology is applicable in high-risk pregnancies.

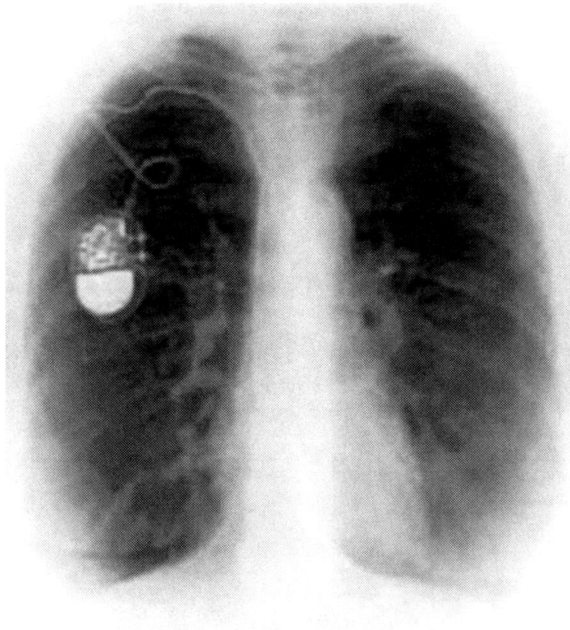

FIGURE 2.23 Pacemaker X-ray. (From Kashi 2007, courtesy of Measurement Specialties, Inc.)

Silicon MEMS-based pressure sensors can be used in intrauterine sensors to measure contraction pressure and frequency during childbirth.[24] An intrauterine pressure sensor is shown in Fig. 2.24.

These disposable sensors are inserted through the uterus and when the baby is ready to be delivered, the sensor is removed.

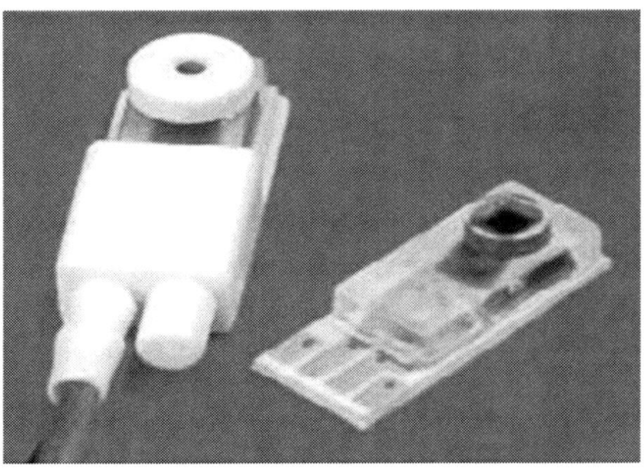

FIGURE 2.24 Intrauterine pressure sensor. (From Kashi 2007, courtesy of Measurement Specialties, Inc.)

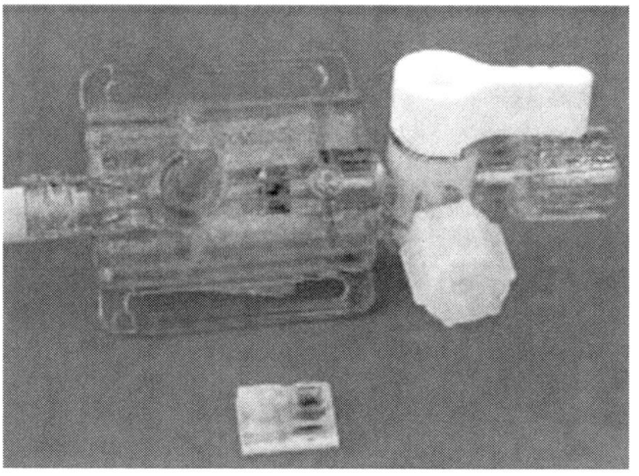

Figure 2.25 Disposable blood pressure sensor. (From Kashi 2007, courtesy of Measurement Specialties, Inc.)

2.4.3 External Sensors Exposed to Body Fluids

Disposable blood pressure sensors, of which one is shown in Fig. 2.25, are an example of external sensors in contact with body fluids. These sensors monitor the blood pressure of the patient continuously and are used in surgical procedures and ICUs.

Another example of sensors exposed to body fluids is the sensor used in the inflation of an angioplasty balloon. Such sensors monitor the pressure applied to inflate the balloon. As medication and body fluids are coming in contact with the sensor, a silicone gel barrier is used to isolate the rest of the sensor.[24]

2.4.4 Sensors Used for External Applications

In some external applications, sensors do not come into contact with either medication or body fluids. These sensors can be used in hospital or home care applications and examples include:[24]

- Magnetic encoders used in syringe pumps to detect flow rate, empty syringe, and occlusion.
- Extremely small MEMS-based accelerometers to study tremors in patients with Parkinson's disease.
- Piezoelectric (and pyroelectric) sensors for sleep apnea study.
- MEMS-based flow sensors used in spirometers to measure breathing strength of asthmatic patients.
- MEMS pressure sensor array to monitor and measure the arterial pressures in the wrist.
- Load cells for infusion pumps that detect occlusion (Fig. 2.26).
- NTC temperature sensors to measure skin or body temperature (Fig. 2.27).

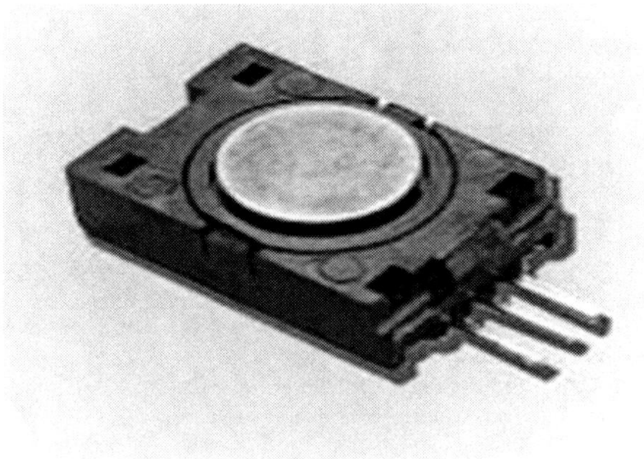

FIGURE 2.26 Infusion pump load cell to detect occlusion. (From Kashi 2007, courtesy of Measurement Specialties, Inc.)

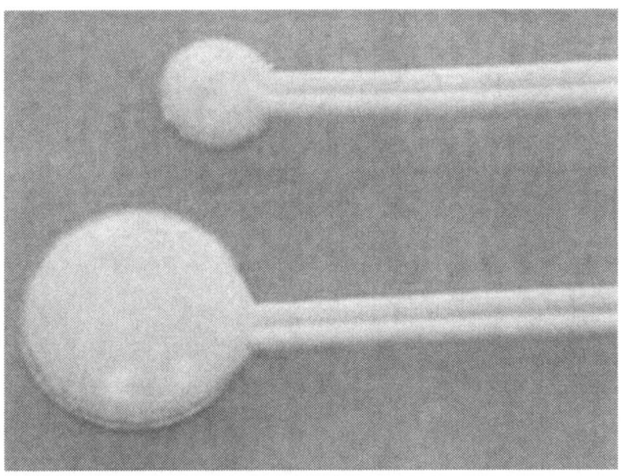

FIGURE 2.27 Reusable NTC thermistor used to measure skin or body temperature. (From Kashi 2007, courtesy of Measurement Specialties, Inc.)

References

1. R. H. Bishop (Ed.). *The Mechatronics Hand Book*, CRC Press, 2002.
2. I. R. Sinclair. *Sensors and Transducers*, 3d ed., Newnes, 2001.
3. J. Fraden. *Hand Book of Modern Sensors-Physics, Designs, and Applications*, 3d ed., Springer, 2004.
4. C. F. Coombs. *Electronic Instrument Hand Book*, 3d ed., McGraw-Hill, USA, 2000.
5. S. Najarian, J. Dargahi, and A. Abouei Mehrizi. *Artificial Tactile Sensing in Biomedical Engineering*, McGraw-Hill, USA, 2009.
6. V. Rajendarn. *Engineering Physics*, Tata McGraw-Hill, New Delhi, 2009.
7. J. G. Webster. *Tactile Sensors for Robotics and Medicine*, John Wiley & Sons, Inc., 1988.

8. G. Gautschi. *Piezoelectric Sensorics: Force, Strain, Pressure, Acceleration and Acoustic Emission Sensors, Materials and Amplifiers*, Springer, 2002.
9. J. S. Wilson. *Sensor Technology Handbook*, Elsevier Inc., 2005.
10. R. Perez. *Design of Medical Electronic Devices*, Academic Press, 2001.
11. J. G. Webster. *The Measurement, Instrumentation, and Sensors Handbook*, CRC Press, 1999.
12. D. S. Nyce. *Linear Position Sensors Theory and Application*, John Wiley & Sons, Inc., 2004.
13. J. J. Carr. *Sensors and Circuits: Sensors, Transducers, and Supporting Circuits for Electronic Instrumentation, Measurement, and Control*, Prentice Hall, 1993.
14. R. A. Russell. *Robot Tactile Sensing*, Prentice-Hall, 1990.
15. T. R. Kurfess (Ed.). *Robotics and Automation Hand Book*, CRC Press, 2005.
16. P. E. Sandin. *Robot Mechanisms and Mechanical Devices Illustrated*, McGraw-Hill, USA, 2003.
17. G. C. Onwubolu. *Mechatronics Principles and Applications*, Elsevier Butterworth-Heinemann, 2005.
18. A. H. Slocum. *Precision Machine Design*, SME, 1992.
19. J. A. Smith, B. J. Polk, T. Kikas, and D. M. Levermore. ChemFETs: Chemical sensors for the real world. www.bizoki.chemistry.gatech.edu/janata-chemicalsensors, 2000.
20. A. S. Dewa and W. H. Ko. "Biosensors." In: *Semiconductor Sensors*, John Wiley & Sons, Inc., 1994, pp. 415–472.
21. M. Graves and B. G. Batchelor (Eds.). *Machine Vision for the Inspection of Natural Products*, Springer, 2003.
22. A. Hornberg (Ed.). *Handbook of Machine Vision*, Wiley-VCH, 2006.
23. R. Jain, R. Kasturi, and B. G. Schunck. *Machine Vision*, McGraw-Hill, USA, 1995.
24. B. Kashi. *Choosing Sensors for Medical Applications*, Measurement Specialties, Inc., 2007.

CHAPTER 3

Actuators and Feedback Sensors

3.1 Introduction

An actuator is any output device, such as an electric motor, that converts energy from an external source into controllable mechanical energy.[1,2] A sensor is an input device which, generally, converts an electrical signal into nonelectrical energy.[3] For example, in an automatic door, a sensor detects motion and sends a signal to an actuator that moves the door. Therefore, because the output from an actuator provides motion or action, they are useful in moving loads and physical objects in any mechatronics system. Furthermore, in conjunction with some form of control device, it can be ensured that they operate to required set points. The type of input supplied to any actuator depends upon the type of actuator.[4] For example, electrical actuators operate using a voltage supply whereas hydraulic actuators operate using liquid flow or pressure.

In this chapter, electromechanical actuators and fluid/compressed gas power actuators are explained, followed by an explanation of other types of actuators such as chemical, shape memory alloy (SMA), ionic polymer-metal composite (IPMC), and microelectromechanical system (MEMS). Although not as common as the aforementioned power actuators, they are still being developed and used in biomedical applications. A brief description on feedback sensors, as well as the criteria for actuator selection, is also given in this chapter.

3.2 Electromechanical Actuators

Electromechanical actuators convert electrical or magnetic energy into mechanical energy. Electromechanical energy conversion occurs in an air gap which separates the moving part and the stationary part of the actuator. There are three types of electromechanical actuators, namely, electromagnetic, electrostatic, and piezoelectric.[5] Electrostatic and piezoelectric actuators make direct use of electrical energy, without the need of using magnetic energy, whereas electromagnetic actuators use magnetic energy to generate force and torque.[4]

Electrostatic transduction, which can be considered as a variable capacitance type, is mostly used when designing multicomponent microactuators. This is because they operate in an analogous mode to variable reluctance type electromagnetic actuators such as variable reluctance stepper motors.[6] Electromagnetic energy conversion is the most common method used in electromechanical actuators because the energy density in magnetic fields is higher than the energy density in electric fields. In magnetic fields, the amount of energy per unit volume of air gap can be five orders of magnitude higher than that of electric fields.[6]

Electromagnetic actuators are those that operate using electricity. These include electric motors, DC motors, solenoids, stepper motors, servomotors, and piezoelectric actuators. The following five sections contain an explanation and description of the construction and operation of these actuators.

3.2.1 Electric Motors

The electric motor was first built by Michael Faraday in 1831. Electric motors are the most common electromechanical actuators and can be classified according to different criteria, such as the type of input required and the method of generating the magnetic field. Electric motors operate using either direct current (DC) or alternating current (AC) and the method of generating the magnetic field is accomplished by using permanent magnets, electromagnets, or induction principles.[4]

An electric motor is composed of a stator and a rotor. The stator is a fixed outer or inner housing of the motor. It supports the material that produces the magnetic field and can be composed of permanent magnet or coil windings. The part that produces the magnetic flux within the stator is the field coil. The moving part of this motor is the rotor which comprises a permanent magnet (or a ferromagnetic core) with coil windings that allows the armature field to interact with the stator field and generate the torque. The armature is the current-carrying winding of the rotor that induces a rotary magnetic field. There is a small gap between the stator and rotor called the air gap in which the magnetic fields interact and generate the output torque.

Most electric motors operate on the principle of induction. When an electric current flows through a wire, a magnetic field is produced around it. Conversely, when a charged coil of wire is placed in an existing magnetic field, the coil will be attracted by one magnet and repelled by the other. The attraction or repulsion of the coil is proportional to the magnetic field created by the current flowing through it. The coil is placed on a spinning shaft in the middle of the motor and is, alternately, attracted by one magnet and repelled by another thereby providing the coil with a circular motion. This is the principle of operation of inductive loads. When a magnetic field is induced by current flowing through a wire, it attracts or repels a magnetic body and when a wire is spinning in a magnetic field, current flow is induced in the wire. When a motor is turned off, a current is generated by virtue of the fact the coil, by inertia, is still spinning in a magnetic field. This current, however, flows in the reverse direction of the current created to run the motor and is called blowback (or back voltage) which can be harmful for the motor's electronics, and a diode is required in line with the motor in order to protect it.[7]

3.2.2 DC Motors

DC motors are very simple and have many applications. DC motors can spin very quickly, at several thousand revolutions per minute (rpm), and possess various speed/torque characteristics that can be changed to match any required application. The speed/torque characteristics of electric motors can be changed by applying external power converters and advanced control methods.

A DC motor has two terminals upon each of which either a positive DC voltage or negative DC voltage connection can be made. When a positive DC voltage is applied to one terminal, and a negative DC voltage to the other, the motor will rotate in one direction; conversely, by reversing the polarity of the connection on each terminal, the motor will spin in the opposite direction.

DC motors can be categorized into two types: brush and brushless. Brush motors consist of an armature and commutator and have conductive brushes which are used for mechanical commutation. The armature is a rotating set of wound wire coils that acts as an electromagnet with two poles; the commutator is a mechanical rotary switch that is in contact with the brushes and also is attached to the rotor shaft. The commutator consists of individual sections (of which there are as many as there are poles on the rotor) and the rotor windings are connected to these sections. The commutator reverses the armature current direction causing the poles of the armature electromagnet to push and pull against the permanent magnets on the outside of the motor. When the poles of the armature electromagnet pass the poles of the permanent magnets, the commutator changes the polarity of the electromagnet and, because the polarity changes instantaneously, it is inertia alone that keeps the motor rotating in the proper direction. Some DC brush motors have multiple poles in their rotors to smooth-out the motion and increase torque.[8] A typical DC brush motor is shown in Fig. 3.1. This particular motor has two poles and uses a permanent magnet.

Brush-type DC servomotors usually consist of an iron core rotor and disk- or cup-type armatures. Servomotors containing a disk-type armature mounted in a pancake-frame motor have a mass that is concentrated close to the motor's faceplate. This permits a short, flat cylindrical housing that enables this type of motor to be mounted in an area where space is limited.[9] Although brush-type DC motors with cup-type armatures have lower weight and inertia than conventional DC servomotors, their drawback is the restriction on their duty cycles. This is because these encapsulated armatures cannot dissipate heat build up as easily as iron core armatures and may become damaged or even destroyed if overheated.[9]

Instead of mechanical commutators and brushes, brushless motors employ electronic commutation systems. A typical brushless motor consists of a permanent magnet rotor, three-phase driving coils, Hall-effect sensors (to provide information on the rotor shaft position), and drive electronics. A typical DC brushless motor is shown in Fig. 3.2.

In order that the polarity of current in the stator windings changes accordingly, the position of the rotor must be determined. This is accomplished by using Hall-effect sensors to detect the position of the rotor. These sensors then send signals to the drive electronics which excite the stator coils at each consecutive phase.

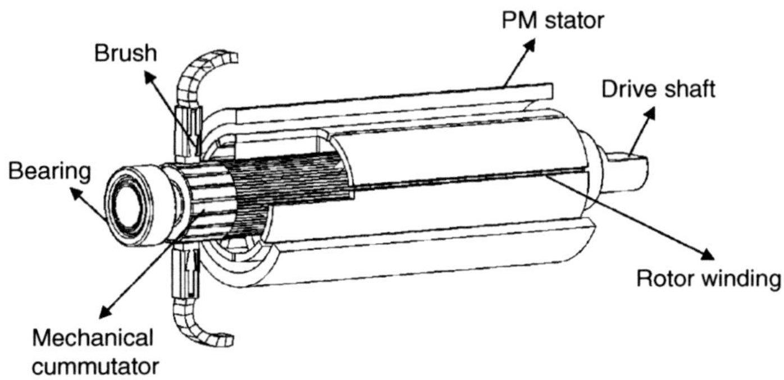

Figure 3.1 Typical DC brush motor.

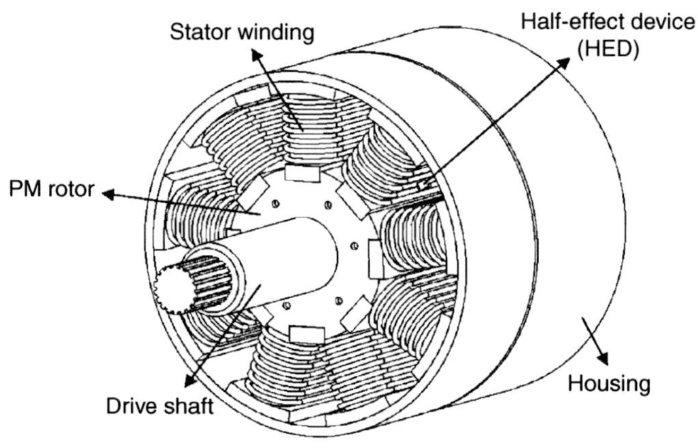

Figure 3.2 Typical DC brushless motor.

The brushless motor can be described as being a form of AC machine with positional feedback.[6] DC brushless motors have various advantages over DC brush motors such as their higher speed capability (due to having no mechanical commutator), greater efficiency (due to more quickly dissipating the stator coil's heat through the motor case), and less maintenance (due to there being no need for periodic brush replacement).[8]

3.2.3 Solenoids

A solenoid is an electromechanical actuator that converts electrical energy into linear or rotary motion. A solenoid consists of a stationary iron or steel frame (stator), a coil, and a ferromagnetic plunger in the center of the coil. A typical solenoid is shown in Fig. 3.3.

Solenoid actuators, and their principle of operation, are very simple. When power from any electrical source goes around the electromagnet, a magnetic field is induced inside the coil. This causes the plunger to move, which increases the flux linkage by closing the air gap between the plunger and the stationary frame. Solenoids can be pull type or push type. When energized, linear solenoids generally pull the plunger into the

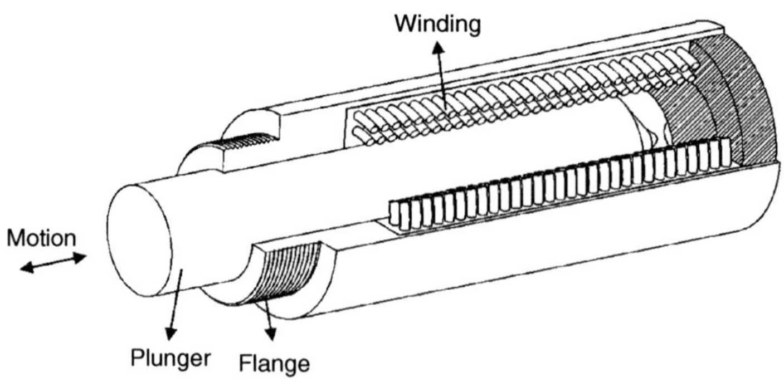

Figure 3.3 Typical solenoid.

coil but in push-type solenoids, the plunger extends through a hole in the back-stop. Therefore, when the coil is energized, the plunger is still pulled into the coil, but is extended by a pushing motion from the back end of the solenoid. By stopping the electric current, the plunger is released and the compression spring sends it back to its initial position with significant force. Return motion can be provided by the weight of the load and/or by using a return spring.

Rotary solenoids operate in a similar fashion to linear solenoids except that their input electrical energy is converted into a rotary, or twisting motion, rather than a linear motion. Rotary actuators are used when controlled speed is a requirement during a rotary stroke application.

When designing and selecting solenoids, major considerations are: force, stroke, temperature, and duty cycle.[6] Here, force is the load developed by the plunger when the coil is energized and stroke is the distance that the plunger moves before it is stopped. The force is dependent upon the stroke and the longer the stroke, the smaller the force. The relationship between the force and the stroke for any particular solenoid is shown by its characteristic curve and is related to the design of some internal parts of the solenoids.

The maximum operating temperature for a solenoid is limited by the rated temperature of the insulating material used in the winding. When the coil is energized, a certain amount of heat is generated and this increases both the temperature and resistance of the coil winding which, in turn, causes a decrease in the current and force output.

The duty cycle is defined as the percentage of on-time to the total time (one complete on/off time) for any one cycle of operation. Solenoids are often classified as those operating under continuous duty cycles and those operating under intermittent duty cycles.[6] Higher performance is obtained in solenoids with higher input power, but extra heat will also be generated so, in order to decrease this, solenoids can be used that operate under intermittent duty cycles (solenoids operating in on/off intervals).

A solenoid valve is an integrated electromechanical device that can actuate a pneumatic valve, a hydraulic valve, or a solenoid switch for use in any application in which a sudden burst of power is required to move any specific part. In medical applications, solenoids must be reliable and highly accurate in terms of force and stroke. For example, in a machine that supplies doses of medicine, the rate of stroke and the force profile of the dosing solenoid are very important to ensure that the correct amount is administered.

3.2.4 Stepper Motors

Stepper motors are electromechanical actuators that convert electrical pulse inputs into mechanical movement. A stepper motor does not rotate continuously but, rather, moves in discrete steps or increments. In rotary stepper motors (which are more common than linear stepper motors), each step equals to a set number of degrees of rotation. The speed of the motor shaft rotation is proportional to the frequency of the input electrical pulses and the length of rotation is proportional to the number of applied electrical pulse inputs.

A stepper motor is controlled by a series of electromagnetic coils. A series of magnets are mounted on the center shaft of the stepper motor and the coils surrounding the shaft are alternately supplied with current or deprived of current. This generates magnetic fields which causes the motor to rotate by repulsing or attracting the magnets on the shaft. A stepper motor has no commutator but, instead, has five or six wires coming

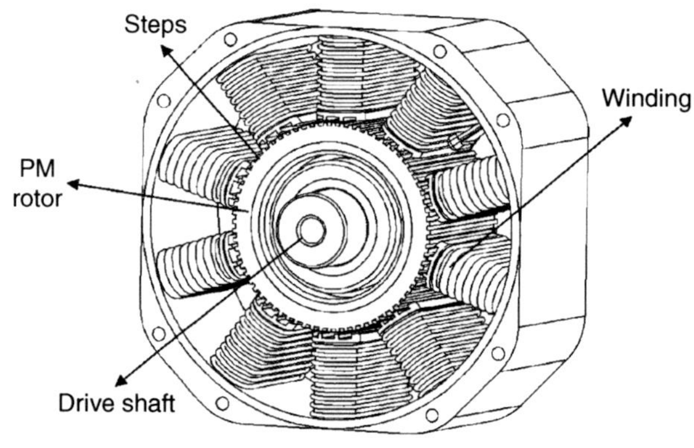

FIGURE 3.4 Typical stepper motor.

out of the motor—one wire for each coil and one or two ground wires. In order for the motor to rotate, power must be applied to one coil after another in the appropriate sequence. A typical stepper motor is shown in Fig. 3.4.

A stepper motor is applicable whenever controlled movement is required. Stepper motors can perform accurate positioning in simple open-loop control systems when they act at low acceleration rates with static loads. They must, however, act in a closed loop with a positioning sensor when higher acceleration values are needed for driving variable loads.[9] A common feature of stepper motor drives is micro-stepping that adjusts the amount of current applied to each phase and permits each full step to be subdivided into smaller steps to permit smoother motion.[8]

The three basic types of stepper motor are: permanent magnet, variable reluctance, and hybrid. Permanent magnet stepper motors have permanent magnets added to their motor structure. The rotor has no teeth but, instead, is magnetized with alternating north and south poles placed in a straight line parallel to the rotor shaft. These magnetized rotor poles provide an increased magnetic flux intensity. Variable reluctance stepper motors have a stator which is similar to the permanent magnet stepper motor except that their rotor is made of soft iron, rather than a permanent magnet, and also has multiple teeth. The poles become magnetized when the stator windings are energized with direct current and rotation occurs when the rotor teeth are attracted to the energized stator poles. Hybrid stepper motors combine the best features of both the permanent magnet and variable reluctance stepper motors. They also have a rotor, with teeth, together with an axially magnetized cylindrical magnet which is concentric to the shaft.

Stepper motors have various advantages, such as being simple to control, their speed is independent of the torque applied on the axis, and the available speed range is greater.[7] Stepper motors produce very little heat when idle so are, therefore, suitable for many different instrument drive motor applications that have limited power.[9]

3.2.5 Servomotor

A common type of servomotor consists of a DC motor, a gear reduction unit, a position-sensing device (e.g., pulse encoder), and a control circuit. A servosystem, in which most servomotors are used, is a closed-loop motion control system which employs one or more feedback loops that continuously compare the system's response with the input commands or settings in order to correct errors in position, speed or torque of motor,

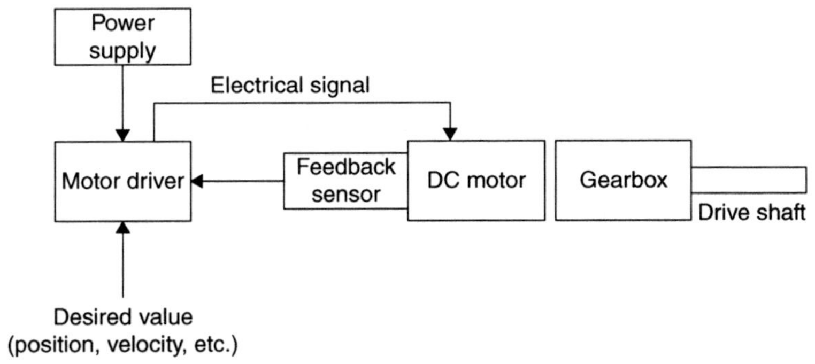

Figure 3.5 A typical block diagram of a servomotor.

and/or load. A servomotor in such a system, therefore, requires its own feedback sensors such as encoders, resolvers, or tachometers.

A typical block diagram of a servomotor is shown in Fig. 3.5 in which the frontal shaft of a DC motor is attached to a gearbox and the rearward shaft is attached to a feedback sensor. The gearbox, which is connected to the main output through the drive shaft, operates as a reduction unit that reduces the speed of the motor. The feedback sensor used in a servomotor is usually an optical pulse encoder. According to the desired value in the system (position, velocity, etc.), the motor driver sends an electrical signal to the motor and receives a response signal from the feedback sensor. The input signal is compared with the feedback signal and the errors are detected. The motor driver then makes proper modifications to the input signal and corrects any errors by ensuring that the servomotor operates within the closed-loop system.

3.2.6 Piezoelectric Actuators

Piezoelectricity is the property inherent within certain types of crystals. It causes an electrical charge in the crystal when exposed to mechanical stress and, conversely, causes physical deformation in the crystal when it is exposed to an electric field.

Piezoelectric actuators convert electrical energy into mechanical displacement or stress, using the piezoelectric effect. Piezoelectric actuators are mainly piezocrystals with two conducting films on the top and bottom. When an electric voltage is applied across the conducting films, the piezocrystal becomes larger in the transverse direction and, when the electric voltage is applied in the opposite direction, the piezocrystal becomes smaller. Piezoelectric actuators can control accurate mechanical displacements and, because they are compact and have no moving parts, are ideally suited for micro and nanoactuation applications.[6] Although piezoelectric actuators have high mechanical durability, and can generate high forces, their disadvantage is that a high voltage is required to drive them.

3.3 Fluid and Pneumatic Power Actuators

A fluid power actuator converts fluid power (pressure and flow-rate) into mechanical work. In general, pressure is controlled for instances in which it is required to determine force or torque whereas the flow-rate is controlled for cases in which it is required to determine kinematic quantities such as position, speed, and acceleration.[6] Power actuators are generally classified according to the type of working medium used. Hydraulic actuators use an incompressible liquid whereas pneumatic actuators use a compressible gas.

Fluid actuators are continuous systems that can measure the positioning of the moveable part of the system at any point in the stroke. They can provide either linear motions (cylinders) or rotational motions (motors). When reciprocating movements are required, with positioning of the actuator at the end of its stroke, two-position or three-position distributor valves with digital operation must be used. On the other hand, when it is necessary to have continual control over positional and transmitted forces in a system, continuous devices must be used. These include proportional valves and servo valves, which are not digital, or digital devices operating with control signal modulation such as the pulse width modulation (PWM) type.[6] A fluid damping system consists of a cylinder which has a steel piston, a piston rod, and a cylinder barrel set-up to convey the damping effect. When fluid/compressed gas moves into the cylinder, it pushes the piston up or down through the length of the cylinder. Cylinders can be classified as being either single acting or double acting. Single-acting cylinders only permit a single work stroke and the fluid pressure is applied on the surface of the piston only in one direction. The external force applied to the rod, or the spring mechanism of the actuator, provides the retract stroke and brings the piston back to its original position. Double-acting cylinders permit both an extend stroke and retract stroke and the fluid acts on both faces of the piston alternately to create both strokes. A double-acting cylinder consists of a tube, which is closed at each end by two heads, and a piston moving inside the barrel carrying the rod connected to the external load. The cylinder is divided into two chambers by the piston. When fluid/compressed gas is sent to one of the chambers through the heads, a pressure difference is created between the two surfaces of the piston and the rod is pushed to the outside discharging the fluid/compressed gas from the other chamber. On the return stroke, the chamber just discharged is filled with fluid/compressed gas and the other chamber is discharged.

Fluid/compressed gas actuation devices have many advantages over electric actuation devices when continuous control of force or speed is a requirement. These include the possibility of maintaining the system under load with no limitation, nor the need for any control devices. Other advantages include performing linear movements directly at high speeds, without the need for devices to convert rotary motion to linear motion. They have higher bandwidths, especially hydraulic systems, and have limited dimensions and therefore low inertia.[6] In the following two sections, hydraulic actuators and pneumatic actuators are explained.

3.3.1 Hydraulic Actuators

A hydraulic actuator creates mechanical movement by controlling an incompressible liquid flow or pressure. The incompressibility of the liquid used in hydraulic actuators helps in positive action or motion, and faster response, while pneumatic systems have longer time delays.[7] An example of a hydraulic actuator is a hydraulic car jack. A hydraulic actuation system generally consists of a pump (which converts input electrical power to hydraulic pressure), an actuator (for converting fluid power into mechanical energy), incompressible fluid (that transfers power in the system), valves (for regulating fluid direction, flow, and pressure), hoses or piping (for transporting fluid in the system) together with filters, accumulator, reservoirs, sensors, and control devices. The pumps used in hydraulic actuators are generally positive displacement pumps

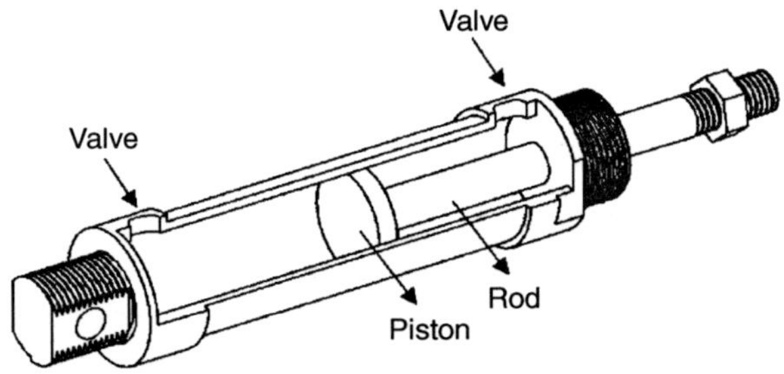

FIGURE 3.6 Schematic of a typical hydraulic actuator.

such as rotary vane, gear, and piston type pumps. Various valves can be used in hydraulic actuators such as check valves, directional valves, flow regulator valves, pressure regulator valves, and servo or proportional valves.

Because the physical displacement of hydraulic actuators is only along the axis of the rod connected to their piston, hydraulic actuators are sometimes required to support loads which are not applied along the axis of the rod so they may become damaged. A schematic of a typical hydraulic actuator is shown in Fig. 3.6.

Hydraulic actuators are applicable to many engineering fields. They are suitable for positioning, forceful applications, velocity control and can be used as either joint or leg actuators in robotics applications in which high payload lifting capability is required.[8] They have various advantages, such as very good force and work densities (more than any other actuator), the ability to perform strokes as long as necessary (if enough fluid is provided), are easily controllable, and do not consume significant power when suspending a payload. They also allow its mechanical damping properties to be incorporated into the system design, and its power source can be located far away from the actuator (although not as far as with electromagnetic actuators).[4,8]

Hydraulic actuators do, however, have certain disadvantages. These include safety problems caused by the high pressures required (which is, however, also one of its advantages), leakage flow (that can become a major problem for actuator performance, safety conditions, and environmental issues), and the inflammability of the oil used.[4]

3.3.2 Pneumatic Actuators

Pneumatic actuators, or pneumatic cylinders, are similar to hydraulic actuators except that they use compressed gas (usually air) instead of a liquid in order to provide pressure. In a pneumatic actuator, a compressible gas is used to create mechanical output motion.[7]

A pneumatic actuation system generally consists of a compressor (which converts electrical input power to air pressure), a compressed air treatment unit (consisting of filters and pressure regulators), valves (for regulating pneumatic power), an actuator (for converting pneumatic power into output mechanical power), hoses or piping (for transporting air into the system) together with sensors and other control devices. Pumps used in pneumatic compressors can be both positive displacement pumps, such as piston and rotary vane pumps that displace the same amount of liquid for each rotating cycle of the pumping element, and non-positive displacement pumps, such as axial and centrifugal pumps that produce continuous flow. The valves used in pneumatic actuation systems to control the air flow are similar to those used in hydraulic actuation systems described in the previous section.

Pneumatic actuators can be applied to robotic industrial grippers and also in medical applications. The advantages of pneumatic actuators are they provide good force and work densities (although not as high as hydraulic actuators), the ability to perform strokes as long as required like their hydraulic counterparts, are easily controllable, and their whole mechanism can be sterilized (including the actuator which makes it suitable for being applied in medical systems). Pneumatic actuators also work at higher temperatures than hydraulic actuators, they operate at a lower working pressure (making them lighter than hydraulic actuators), and have less complex parts because exhausted pressurized air in the actuator can be released to the environment through an outlet valve rather than being sent through a return line.[4,8,10] Another advantage with pneumatic actuators is that air is easily available and no recycling is necessary. Air is nonflammable and so any leakage does not threaten the safety of the system, and its viscosity, which controls the systems performance, changes negligibly.[7] Furthermore, the power source providing the energy can be located far away from the actuator.

The disadvantage of pneumatic actuators compared with hydraulic actuators are they cannot operate at high pressures because of the high compressibility of the gases, they are slower and less stiff against perturbations, they are less efficient because of the losses of energy due to the heat transfer (in the air cooling), are more prone to leakage, and require lubrication.[4]

3.4 Other Actuators

Because the majority of robotic and automated mechanical systems use electric and power (fluid/compressed gas) actuators, these two main types are referred to as conventional actuators. Recently, however, advances in smart-material technology have introduced lightweight and strong materials which can be used to develop novel actuators. Unlike conventional actuators, smart-material actuators can be embedded in a distributed manner and integrated into load-bearing structures that could be used to suppress vibration, cancel noise, and change shape.[6] Two common examples of these actuators are shape memory alloy (SMA) and ionic polymer-metal composite (IPMC) actuators which are explained in this section as are chemical and MEMS actuators. Although none of these actuators are as common as electrical and fluid power actuators, they are being especially developed for use in medical fields.

3.4.1 Chemical Actuators

A good example of chemical actuators is hydrogels. Polymer hydrogels are hydrophilic materials with three-dimensional polymeric networks that can absorb large quantities of water without dissolving. Polymer hydrogels exhibit great size and shape changes in response to various environmental stimuli, such as temperature, pH, solvent, and electric field.

Hydrogels can be used as actuators in bioMEMS devices due to their shape changes, and as artificial muscles due to their great changes in physical dimensions caused by changes in the polarity of the electric field.[11]

Thin hydrogel films can be applicable as microfluidic devices for sensors and actuators. Automatic microfluidic systems, based on the sensor-actuator properties of hydrogels, and can perform unique functions compared with other systems or actuators and can be applied to hydrodynamic transistors, micropumps, and tunable microlenses.[12]

3.4.2 Shape Memory Alloy Actuators

Shape memory alloys (SMAs) are active materials that can return to a predetermined shape or size when heated. The most common type of shape memory alloys is nickel-titanium alloy, called Nitinol. It has very good electrical and mechanical properties, long fatigue life, and high corrosion resistance.[13]

The principle of operation of SMAs is that when they are cooled below a critical temperature, their crystal structure goes into a martensitic phase and, when heated above the critical temperature, goes into an austenitic phase. This means that SMAs have the capability of returning to their original shape when heated up and have a phase change from martensitic to austenitic structure, hence generating high forces. So, SMAs can be used as an actuator when they are operated above the critical temperature.

SMA actuators are used in a wide range of applications including robotics, medical equipment, and the aerospace industry. Many of the current applications of SMAs have been used in the biomedical area including orthodontic, orthopedic, cardiovascular, and surgical applications. For example, SMAs can be used in a wide variety of medical devices such as dental arches, spinal vertebra spacers, stents, catheter guide wires, and laparoscopy tools.[14]

Despite the various advantages of SMA actuators including easy miniaturization, high energy density, and flexible configuration, they have some disadvantages including low speed, temperature dependence, and low efficiency.[4]

3.4.3 Ionic Polymer-Metal Composite Actuators

Ionic polymer-metal composites (IPMCs) are smart composites possessing the same characteristics as both actuators and sensors. IPMCs are usually made of Nafion films (provided by Dupont). When strips of these composites are bent, an electric voltage is generated across the thickness of the strip between the two attached conducting electrodes. Therefore, IPMCs act as large motion sensors and, conversely, when an electric field is imposed through the thickness of IPMC strips, they undergo large bending and flapping displacement and so act as large motion actuators.[15]

In biomedical applications, IPMCs are generally used as actuators rather than sensors and operate like biological muscles so are therefore suitable for being used as artificial muscles. IPMC actuators have various advantages compared to other actuators (such as peizocerams or SMAs) including being highly active at lower voltages compared and they also have a significantly higher response time than shape memory alloys. They operate best in a humid environment and, being made as a self-contained encapsulated actuator to operate in dry environments, have the unique characteristic of low weight, high toughness, large actuation strain constant, and inherent vibration damping capability.[15] The disadvantage of IPMCs, and one that limits their application as an actuator, is that they only generate a low actuating force since they are dependent upon the bending stiffness and thickness of the ionic polymer membrane.[16]

3.4.4 MEMS Actuators

Microelectromechanical system (MEMS) actuators are based mostly on electrostatic transduction. The difference between the electrostatic motors and conventional motors is that electrostatic motors are based on electrostatic forces while conventional motors are based on magnetic forces. Although electrostatic forces are appropriate actuating forces for MEMS actuators, electromagnetic actuation is not common at the micro scale compared to the conventional scale.

Some smart solid-state materials such as SMAs, conducting polymers and dielectric elastomers can also be used in microactuators. Although these materials exhibit high strain, thin-film piezoelectric transducer (PZT) is preferred to these actuator materials because of its efficiency, speed (over 100 kHz of bandwidth) and controllability.[17] Microactuator technologies have various characteristics of which some are commonalities with microsensors including repeatability, the ability to be constructed at a small scale, immunity from external effects, sufficient bandwidth and linearity with microactuators including achievable force, power, displacement, bandwidth (or speed of response), and efficiency.[6]

3.5 Feedback Sensors

In a closed-loop motion control system, the system's response is compared continuously with the input signal. Feedback sensors are required in a closed-loop motion control system to correct errors in position, velocity or acceleration of the motor, torque (in rotary actuators), and stroke (in linear actuators). The most common feedback required in a closed-loop motion control system is position feedback. Various kinds of feedback sensors are used in mechatronic systems such as encoders, tachometers, resolvers, linear variable differential transformers (LVDTs), potentiometers, laser interferometers, etc. These sensors are explained in Chap. 2.

Optical encoders are the most common feedback sensor and can produce either sine waves or pulses. Analog encoders generate sine waves and external circuitry is required for counting, but digital encoders contain circuitry for translating sine waves into pulses.[9] Absolute optical encoders can save the last position of the encoder code disk as a binary word and, therefore, can provide precise position information.

Feedback sensor selection is based on an evaluation of various characteristics of the sensor such as the sensor's accuracy, repeatability, ruggedness, temperature limits, size, weight, mounting requirements, and cost, with the relative preference of each one determined by the required application.[9]

3.6 Selection Criteria

Various parameters must be considered for the selection of proper actuators in a mechatronics system. Choosing a specific actuator for use in a mechatronics system depends on the preference of these parameters. Some of the performance parameters required before choosing an actuator for a specific need are: type of required motion (linear or rotational), size and weight of the actuator, power or stroke, speed of reacting to input signals, type of actuator input energy (such as electric, fluid, etc.), limitations in materials selection (e.g., in specific medical applications), limitations of noise-generating for noise-sensitive systems, maintenance and cleaning cost, the amount of heat generated while actuating, controllability, and cost.

References

1. O. Gomis-Bellmunt. "Design, Modeling, Identification and Control of Mechatronic Systems", PhD thesis, Technical University of Catalonia, 2007.
2. O. Gomis-Bellmunt, S. Galceran-Arellano, A. Sudrià-Andreu, D. Montesinos-Miracle, and L. F. Campanile. "Linear Electromagnetic Actuator Modeling for Optimization of Mechatronic and Adaptronic Systems," *Mechatronics*, vol. 17, 2007, pp. 153–163.
3. J. Fraden. *Hand Book of Modern Sensors- Physics, Designs, and Applications*, Springer, 3d ed., 2004.
4. O. Gomis-Bellmunt and L. F. Campanile. *Design Rules for Actuators in Active Mechanical Systems*, Springer, 2010.
5. R. H. Bishop (Ed.). *The Mechatronics Hand Book*, CRC Press, 2002.
6. R. H. Bishop (Ed.). *The Mechatronics Handbook: Mechatronic Systems, Sensors, and Actuators*, 2nd ed., CRC Press, 2008.
7. G. C. Onwubolu. *Mechatronics Principles and Applications*, Elsevier Butterworth-Heinemann, 2005.
8. T. R. Kurfess (Ed.). *Robotics and Automation Hand Book*, CRC Press, 2005.
9. P. E. Sandin. *Robot Mechanisms and Mechanical Devices-Illustrated*, McGraw-Hill, 2003.
10. K. Daeyoung, R. Nakamura, E. Kobayashil, I. Sakuma, and T. Dohi. "Application of Compact Pneumatic Actuators to Laparoscopic Manipulator," *MICCAI 2001;* W. Niessen and M. Viergever (Eds.). Springer-Verlag Berlin Heidelberg, 2001, pp. 1424–1425.
11. K. Park, R.M. Ottenbrite, and T. Okano, (Eds.). *Biomedical Applications of Hydrogels Hand Book*, Springer, 2010.
12. G. Gerlach and K. F. Arndt (Eds.). *Hydrogel Sensors and Actuators*, Springer Series on Chemical Sensors and Biosensors, vol. 6, Springer, 2009.
13. N. P. Mahalik. *Mechatronics Principles, Concepts and Applications*, Tata McGraw-Hill, New Delhi, 2003.
14. L. G. Machado and M. A. Savi. "Medical Applications of Shape Memory Alloys," *Brazilian Journal of Medical and Biological Research*, vol. 36, 2003, pp. 683–691.
15. M. Shahinpoor, Y. Bar-Cohen, T. Xue, J. O. Simpson, and J. Smith. "Ionic Polymer-Metal Composites (IPMC) As Biomimetic Sensors and Actuators," *Proceedings of SPIE's 5th Annual International Symposium on Smart Structures and Materials*, San Diego, 1998.
16. S. J. Lee, M. J. Han, S. J. Kim, J. Y. Jho, H. Y. Lee, and Y. H. Kim. "A New Fabrication Method for IPMC Actuators and Application to Artificial Fingers," *Smart Materials and Structures*, vol. 15, 2006, pp. 1217–1224.
17. N. J. Conway, Z. J. Traina, and S. G. Kim. "A Strain Amplifying Piezoelectric MEMS Actuator," *Journal of Micromechanics and Microengineering*, vol. 17, 2007, pp. 781–787.

CHAPTER 4

Mechanisms and Mechanical Devices

4.1 Introduction

The motion of any rigid body (even a very complex motion) is a combination of translational and rotational motions. A *translational motion* is defined as the movement along one or more of the three coordinate axes, and a *rotational motion* is defined as the rotation about one or more of the coordinate axes. For example, when instructing a robot to carry out a task, the required motion for performing that task must be broken down into translational and rotational motions.

Kinetics is the branch of mechanics that studies the motion of a body or a system of bodies without consideration given to its mass or the forces acting on it. In this branch of classical mechanics, a *mechanism* is defined as being the combination of rigid bodies connected together by joints in order to transmit, control, or constrain,[1] thereby converting motion from one form into another.

Although electric motors that rotate at high speed and low torque are usually adequate for most purposes, in many applications, slow rotation with high torque is required. Reducing the speed of motors by a controller decreases their efficiency and, although stepper motors can be used to solve this problem, they have certain disadvantages such as rough performance at low speeds (unless micro-stepping is used), consuming current regardless of load, limited sizes available, are noisy, torque decreases with speed and can stall or lose position without a control loop.[2] So, to solve this problem, the electric motor can be attached to a mechanism that transforms its high speed and low torque into the low speed and high torque required for most applications in mechatronics.

There are various mechanisms and mechanical devices, including rack and pinions, gears, chains, belt drives, linkages, cams, etc. In this chapter, different types of such devices are described and their function explained. They are classified according to their function and are explained in six categories namely: conversion of rotational motion into linear motion and vice versa, changing rotational speed, torque and the angular orientation of rotational motion, transformation of rotary motion in one plane to another, brakes and clutches, creation of a particular manner of motion, and bearings.

4.2 Conversion of Rotational Motion into Linear Motion and Vice Versa

Conversion of rotational motion into linear motion and also conversion of linear motion into rotational motion is one of the common motion transformations required in mechatronics systems. Common mechanisms to achieve this are rack and pinions, and ball screws.

4.2.1 Rack and Pinion

A rack and pinion, shown in Fig. 4.1, consists of a pair of gears which converts rotational motion into linear motion and linear motion into rotational motion. The pinion is a normal round gear and the rack is straight or flat. Teeth of the rack mesh with the teeth of the pinion gear. When rotational motion is applied to the pinion, it will cause the rack to move to the side.

4.2.2 Ball Screw

A ball screw mechanism, shown in Fig. 4.2, consists of a threaded shaft which provides a helical raceway for ball bearings. The collection of steel balls acts as a nut and the threaded shaft acts as a screw. Ball screws convert rotational motion to linear motion with little friction. Ball screws are made to close tolerances and can provide high precision in various applications. They can be back-driven according to their lead angle and the screw shaft can be driven linearly to rotate the ball nut because there is little friction.

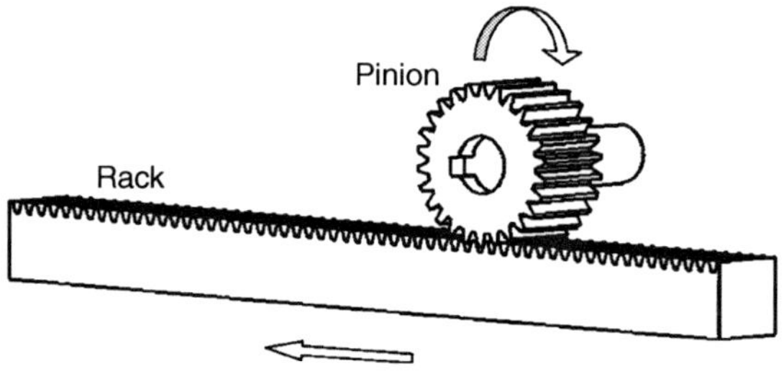

FIGURE 4.1 The rack and pinion.

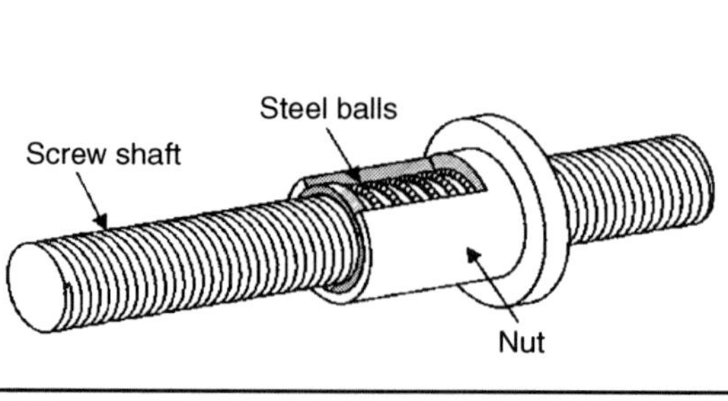

FIGURE 4.2 The ball screw.

4.3 Changing Rotational Speed, Torque, and Angular Orientation of Rotational Motion

A pair of rolling cylinders can be used to transfer rotational motion from one shaft to another and the transfer of motion between the cylinders is related to frictional forces between their contact surfaces. A good way to prevent slip between these cylinders is by adding meshing teeth to them. Here, a pair of meshed gear wheels can be used to transfer rotational motion between two shafts. Gears are versatile mechanical components used for performing various types of power transmission or motion control.[2] They can transmit power and motion between parallel, intersecting, or even skew shafts. Gears with the same tooth size can be used together and transfer very large ratios of power and motion.

The *gear ratio* is defined as the ratio of the angular velocities of a pair of intermeshed gear wheels.[1] The ratio of angular velocities of a pair of intermeshed gear wheels is equal to the inverse ratio of their number of teeth on each wheel as shown in Eq. (4.1):

$$\frac{\omega_1}{\omega_2} = \frac{\text{number of teeth on wheel 2}}{\text{number of teeth on wheel 1}} \tag{4.1}$$

Because the number of teeth on a wheel is proportional to the diameter of the wheel, the ratio of angular velocities of a pair of intermeshed gear wheels is equal to the inverse ratio of their diameters, as shown in Eq. (4.2):

$$\frac{\omega_1}{\omega_2} = \frac{\text{number of teeth on wheel 2}}{\text{number of teeth on wheel 1}} = \frac{d_2}{d_1} \tag{4.2}$$

A set of two or more gears used to transmit torque between two parts is called the gear train. In this section, we explain some common gears including spur gears, bevel gears, face gears, and worm gears together with two common gear trains including epicyclic gear trains and harmonic drive gear trains. These are used to change rotational speed, torque, and the angular orientation of rotational motion.

4.3.1 Gear Terminology

Some common definitions in gear terminology are explained as follows:

Pitch circle: The circle on which spacing or tooth profiles is established and from which the tooth proportions are constructed.

Addendum: The height by which a tooth projects beyond the pitch circle or pitch line.

Dedendum: The distance between the bottom land of the gear tooth and the pitch circle.

Addendum circle: The theoretical circle considered in the outer diameter of the gear.

Dedendum circle: The theoretical circle considered through the bottom lands of the gear.

Clearance: The amount by which the dedendum in a given gear exceeds the addendum of its mating gear.

Circular pitch: The distance along the pitch circle or pitch line between corresponding profiles of adjacent teeth.

Diametral pitch: The ratio of the number of teeth of a gear to the pitch diameter.

Pressure angle: The angle at a pitch point between the line of pressure which is normal to the tooth surface, and the plane tangent to the pitch surface.

Contact ratio: The number of angular pitches through which a tooth surface rotates from the beginning to the end of contact.

Backlash: The amount by which the width of a tooth space exceeds the thickness of the engaging tooth on the pitch circles.

4.3.2 Spur and Helical Gears

A spur gear, shown in Fig. 4.3, is a cylindrical gear that has teeth parallel to the axis of rotation used for the transmission of rotational motion between parallel shafts. A helical gear is similar to a cylindrical gear except that its teeth are at an angle to the axis of rotation (Fig. 4.4). The advantage of helical gears is that they deliver a smoother drive and have a longer life because each individual tooth only becomes gradually engaged. Their disadvantage is the axial force component on the shaft bearing caused by the inclination of the teeth to the axis of rotation. This, however, can be overcome by using double helical teeth.[1]

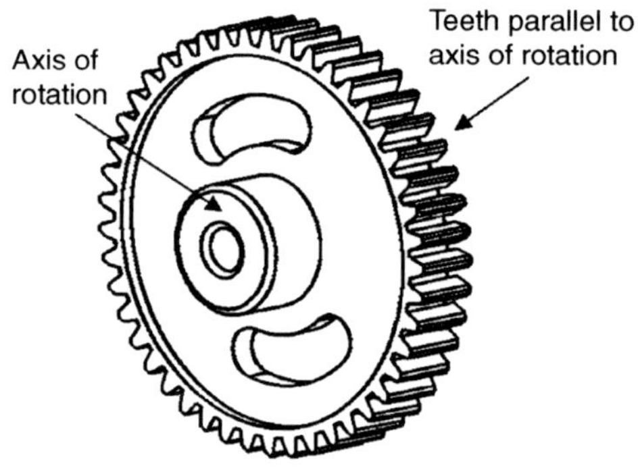

Figure 4.3 The spur gear.

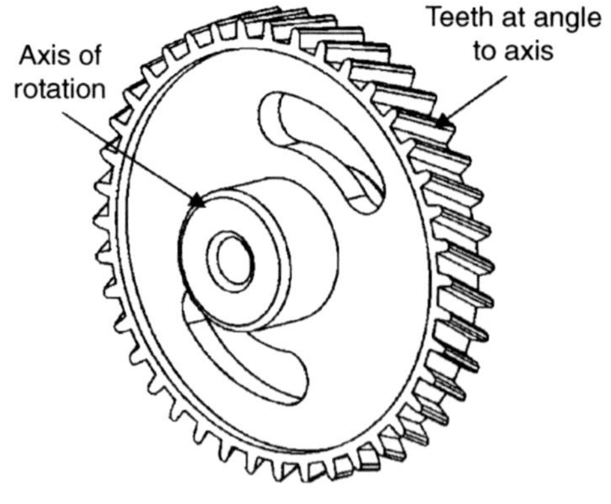

Figure 4.4 The helical gear.

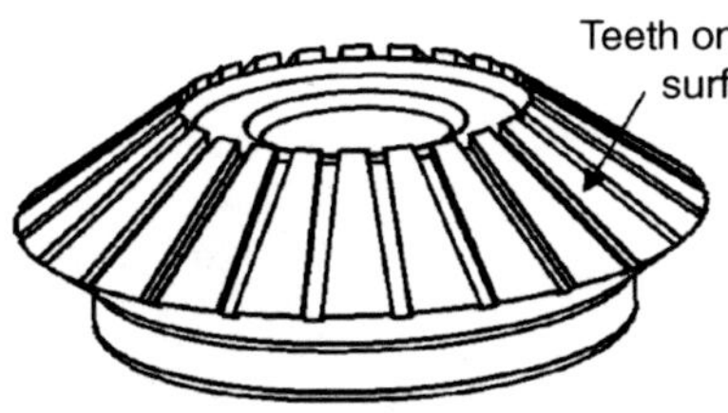

FIGURE 4.5 The bevel gear.

4.3.3 Bevel Gears

A bevel gear, shown in Fig. 4.5, has teeth on a conical surface and is used for the transmission of rotational motion with intersecting axes.

The simplest type of bevel gear is a straight bevel gear. Contact lines of straight bevel gear are parallel to the pitch line and the straight teeth engage with full-line contact. Another type of bevel gear is the spiral bevel gear that has helical teeth which engage gradually with at least two teeth being in contact simultaneously. Spiral bevel gears have lower tooth loading compared to straight bevel gears and they can rotate up to eight times faster.[2]

4.3.4 Face Gears

A face gear, shown in Fig. 4.6, has straight tooth surfaces which are tapered toward the center of the gear. Face gears are used in turning right-angle drives, but they have low load capacities.[2]

4.3.5 Worm Drive

A worm drive, shown in Fig. 4.7, is composed of a worm and a worm gear. The worm acts as a screw and, when it rotates, causes the worm gear also to rotate. Although worm drives are used for reducing rotational speed and transmitting high torque, they can become self-locking in large reduction ratios because they are not back-drivable (the worm gear cannot drive the worm). This important feature of worm gear meshes is called irreversibility which can be useful as a locking mechanism. The disadvantage of worm gears is their low efficiency because, since the worm drives the gear primarily with slipping motion, there are high friction losses.

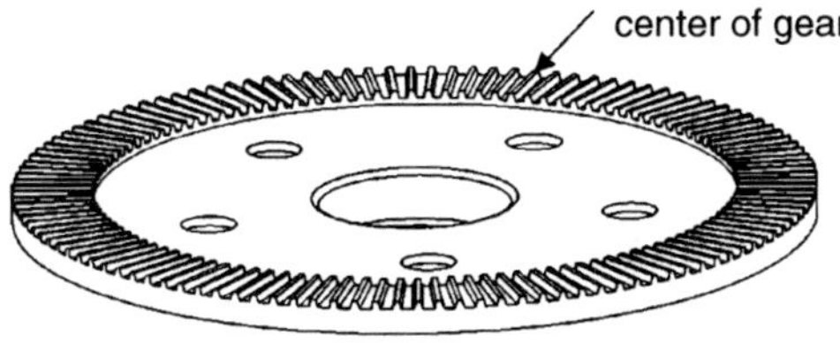

FIGURE 4.6 The face gear.

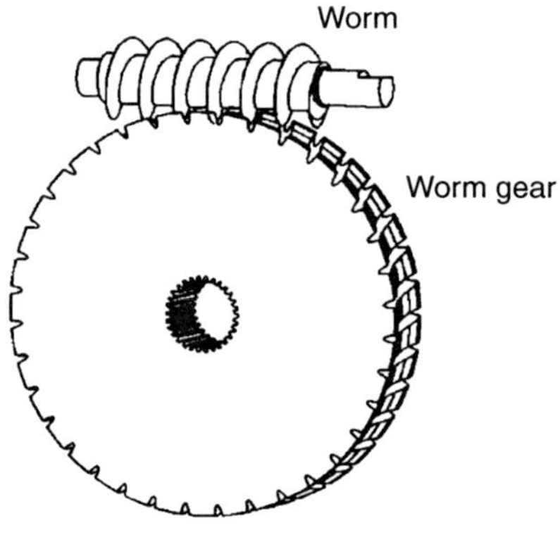

FIGURE 4.7 The worm drive.

4.3.6 Harmonic Drive Gear Train

A harmonic drive gear train, shown in Fig. 4.8, is a special type of mechanical gear system invented in 1957. The harmonic drive gear train can be used in motion-control applications and robotics.[3] It is based on the strain-wave gearing principle, related to the flexibility of metals, and consists of three basic components: a wave generator, a flex spline, and a circular spline.

The wave generator is composed of an elliptical-shaped plug and an outer ball bearing into which the plug is inserted, giving it an elliptical shape. The flex spline is a thin-walled, flexible metal cup with external teeth which are positioned radially on the outside of the flex spline. The flex spline fits tightly over the wave generator so that as the wave generator plug rotates, it conforms to the shape of the plug but does not rotate with the wave generator.

The circular spline is a thick-walled, nonrotating rigid ring with internal teeth. The flex spline and wave generator are located inside the circular spline. The teeth of the elliptical flex spline only engage with the internal teeth of the circular spline in two areas of the flex spline, along the major axis of the ellipse and on opposite sides.

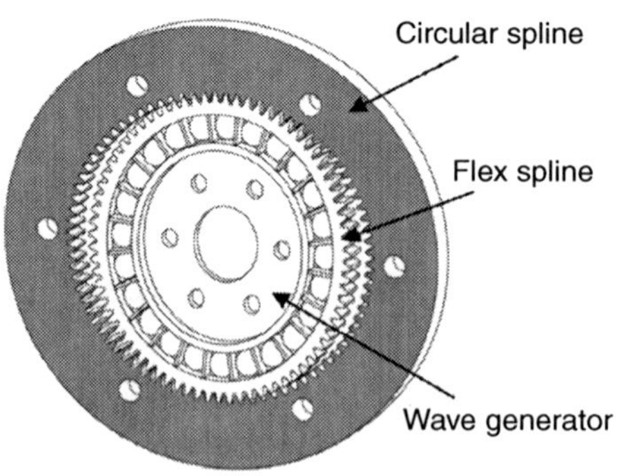

FIGURE 4.8 The harmonic drive gear train.

When the wave generator rotates, it causes the teeth of the flex spline to mesh with the teeth of the circular spline. Because the major axis of the flex spline actually rotates with the wave generator, the points where the teeth mesh with each other revolve around the center point at the same rate as the wave generator. However, because there are typically two or three fewer teeth on the flex spline than there are on the circular spline, it means that for every full revolution of the wave generator, the flex spline does not rotate a complete 360 degrees. Therefore, it rotates more slowly in the fixed circular spline and in the opposite direction compared to the wave generator. In a harmonic drive mechanism, the gearing reduction ratio for one revolution of motion can be written as in Eq. (4.3):

$$\text{Reduction ratio} = \frac{\text{flex spline teeth} - \text{circular spline teeth}}{\text{flex spline teeth}} \tag{4.3}$$

For example, if there are 202 teeth on the circular spline and 200 on the flex spline, the reduction ratio is (200 – 202)/200 = –0.01

The harmonic drive gear train has various advantages, including zero backlash, high reduction ratios, compactness, high efficiency, and excellent repeatability and resolution.[2] However, the disadvantage of the harmonic drive gear train is its torsional windup. The drive's tooth design allows only one tooth to be completely engaged at each end of the major axis of the wave generator but only when there is no torsional load. When the torsional load increases, the teeth bend slightly and the flex spline distorts slightly, allowing adjacent teeth to engage. This bending and distortion causes torsional windup which is one of the main reasons of positional error in harmonic drive gearboxes.[2]

4.3.7 Epicyclic Gear Train

The epicyclic gear train (or planetary gear train) is a gear system consisting of a central gear (sun gear), one or more outer gears (planet gears that revolve around the sun gear), and an outer ring gear (or annulus) which meshes with the planet gears. Typically, the planet gears are held by a carrier which rotates relative to the sun gear. An epicyclic gear train is shown in Fig. 4.9.

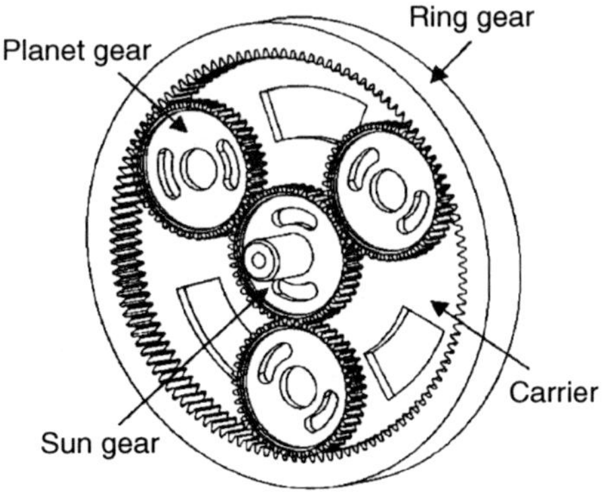

Figure 4.9 The epicyclic gear train.

The ring gear has teeth on the inner rim and, when fixed, is provided with a resilient mount which allows for a certain degree of distortion to occur reducing tooth loading. The planet wheels are located by a planet carrier ring fitted at each end. The system may be constructed in three different modes, namely planetary, star, and solar.

In the planetary mode, the ring wheel is fixed. Input is via the sun wheel and output through the planet wheel carrier ring. In the star mode, the planet wheel carrier is fixed and input is via the sun wheel and output through the ring gear. In the solar mode, the sun gear is fixed, but this system is seldom used except in back-to-back epicyclic systems. In each case, the fixed member is called the torque reaction member and the number of wheels is determined by tooth loading.

4.4 Transformation of Rotary Motion in One Plane to Motion in Another Plane

The transformation of rotary motion from one plane to another, and changing the axis of rotation, can be obtained by direct and indirect methods. Couplings are the most common direct method and belts and chains are the most common indirect method. Each can be used to replace a group of gears, bearings, and shafts and are explained in this section.

4.4.1 Couplings

Couplings are used to connect the ends of two shafts together for the purposes of transmitting motion and power and can allow for some degree of misalignment and/or end movement. Couplings can be either solid or flexible. Solid couplings are used to hold the end of two or more shafts together to make one solid shaft, while flexible couplings are used to join shafts together which are, or might become, slightly out of alignment. Such a coupling is shown in Fig. 4.10.

Solid couplings are used in applications in which precise shaft alignment is needed. They have a very simple design and clamp onto each shaft to convey the torque from one shaft to another.

Flexible couplings are used to transmit torque while allowing for some axial, radial, and angular misalignment. One of the most common flexible couplings is the universal

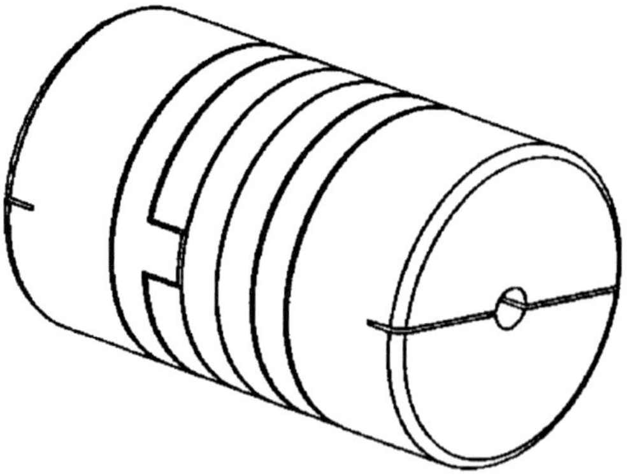

FIGURE 4.10 The flexible coupling.

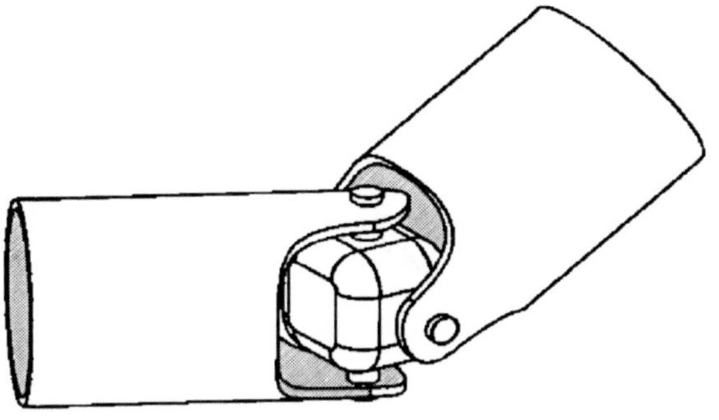

FIGURE 4.11 The universal joint.

joint, or Cardan joint, shown in Fig. 4.11. The universal joint is a joint or coupling in a rigid rod that permits the rod to bend in any direction. It consists of a pair of hinges oriented at 90 degrees to each other and connected by a cross shaft and are used in shafts that transmit rotary motion.

The shaft design at each end of the coupling may be different. For shaped shafts, a coupling with the same shape and size as the shaft is required and, for smooth shafts, the required coupling must clamp to the shaft tight enough to convey the torque through friction with the shaft surface.[2]

4.4.2 Chain

Chain drives, shown in Fig. 4.12, are mechanical devices which can be used to transform rotary motion from one plane to another and are typically constructed of metal.

The roller chain is an efficient power transfer method and is the one mostly used. It consists of steel rollers held together by side links. The roller chain can handle some misalignment between the driver and driven gears and, generally, does not require that any accompanying pulleys be precisely tensioned.[2]

4.4.3 Belt

The belt drive is a method of transmitting power between two shafts especially when the distances between the shafts are large. Belts can handle some misalignment and the

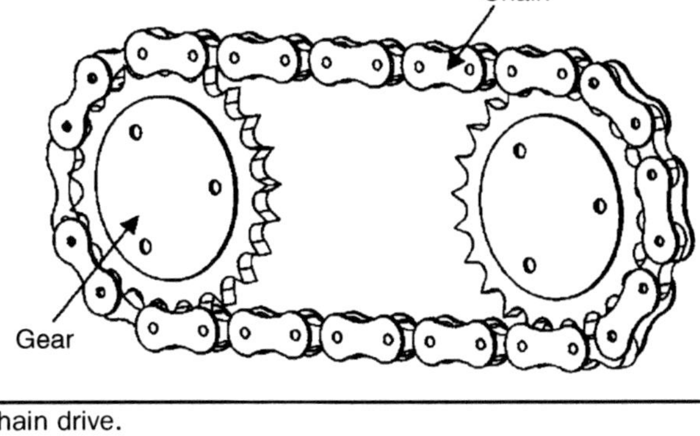

FIGURE 4.12 The chain drive.

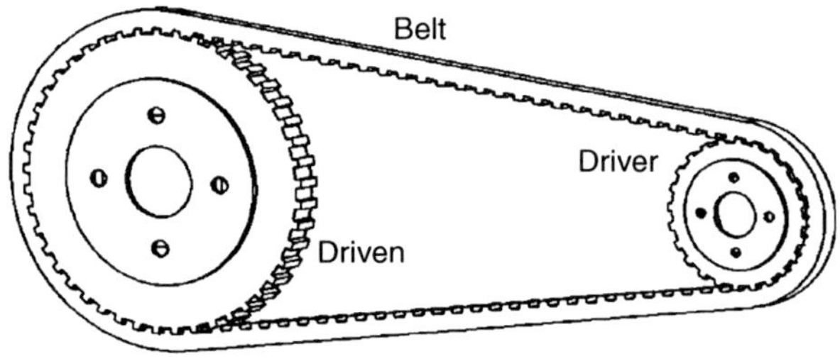

FIGURE 4.13 The timing belt.

advantage of belts is that their length can easily be adjusted to a wide range of shaft-to-shaft distances.

One of the most common types of belts is the timing belt, shown in Fig. 4.13. These are an excellent method of power transfer and solve the slip problem of other types of belts such as flat belts, O-ring belts, V-belts, etc. Timing belts have flexible teeth and the load is distributed over all the teeth in contact with the pulley.

When the belt drive operates under load, a difference develops between the belt tension on the tight side and the slack side of the driver pulley. This difference is called effective tension, T_e, which represents the force transmitted from the driver pulley to the belt.[4] T_e is described in Eq. (4.4):

$$T_e = T_1 - T_2 \tag{4.4}$$

where T_1 and T_2 are the tight and slack side tensions, respectively.

The driving torque, M_T, is given in Eq. (4.5):

$$M_T = T_e \frac{d}{2} \tag{4.5}$$

where d is the pitch diameter of the driver pulley.

4.5 Clutches and Brakes

Clutches and brakes are devices used for effective control and transmission of drive torque, speed, and power in rotating drive systems. Clutches provide transmission of torque and motion from an input shaft to an output shaft, and brakes stop and hold a load. When one component rotates and the other is fixed to a nonrotating reference plane, the device operates as a brake and, when both components rotate, the device operates as a clutch.[5]

Clutches and brakes can be categorized according to their actuating system such as mechanical, electrical, fluid, etc., or according to their technique of operation such as friction, electromagnetic, mechanical lockup, etc.

4.5.1 Brakes

A brake is a mechanical device used for stopping a moving body, or bringing it to a state of uniform motion and holding it against the action of external forces or turning moments.[1]

The energy removed during the process of braking is in the form of heat. Because this generated heat decreases efficiency and causes brake fade (loss of stopping power), it must be dissipated from the system. If the rate of heat generation in the brake becomes more than the rate of heat dissipation, the temperature of the friction material increases and causes a decrease in the coefficient of friction. Hence, for providing the same degree of braking, a greater force must be applied on the brakes.

Mechanical brakes work by mechanical means such as levers, springs, and pedals and, according to the shape of the friction material, they are categorized into block brakes, internal or external shoe brakes, disk brakes, and band brakes.[6] Other types of brakes are hydraulic and pneumatic brakes which use fluid pressure such as oil pressure or air pressure, and electrical brakes which use magnetic forces to stop or hold a load.

4.5.2 Clutches

A clutch is a mechanical device used to connect or disconnect a driven component from a prime mover, such as an engine or motor, and to accelerate a rotating machine from rest to the required speed.[5]

Clutches can be classified by their techniques of operation into positive contact clutches (which transmit power by means of interlocking of jaws or teeth), friction clutches (which transmit power by means of friction between contacting surfaces), electromagnetic clutches (which transmit power by means of magnetic field), and fluid clutches (which transmit power by means of hydraulic pressure).[6]

The most popular type of clutch is the friction clutch which uses the friction developed between two mating surfaces to transmit the power or motion. One surface is metallic, generally cast iron, and the other surface has a friction facing made from molded organic material. Friction clutches come in various types, including cone clutch, disk clutch, centrifugal clutch, etc.

When designing clutches, points to consider include avoiding an excessive amount of actuation force, constant coefficient of friction, dissipation of heat, and limited wear to provide reasonable clutch life.[5]

4.6 Creation of a Particular Manner of Motion

Sometimes, the transformation of one motion, such as rotation, into any other motion is required in a system. Cams and linkages are mechanical devices that can be used to obtain a motion which must be changed in a particular manner.

4.6.1 Cam Mechanism

A cam is a rotating or sliding element which is in contact with another element called the follower and both are placed on a fixed frame. The cam gives a prescribed particular motion to the follower by its oscillating or rotational motion. A typical cam mechanism is shown in Fig. 4.14. As the cam rotates, the profile or shape of the cam causes the follower to rise, dwell, and fall and create a specific motion. Then, the motion of the follower is transmitted to another mechanism or another part of the mechanism.

Cam mechanisms can be classified by the modes of input to output motion, the configuration and arrangement of the follower, the shape of the cam, the different types of motion events of the follower, and the motion characteristics of the cam profile.[1]

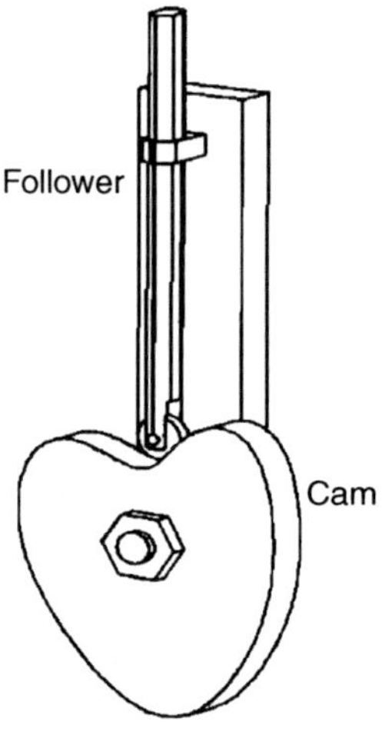

FIGURE 4.14 The cam mechanism.

4.6.2 Linkage

A mechanical linkage is a series of rigid links connected together with joints to form a motion. The joints have various degrees of freedom to allow motion between each link. When two or more links are movable relative to a fixed link, the linkage is called a mechanism. A linkage mechanism is shown in Fig. 4.15.

The simplest closed loop kinematic linkage is the four-bar linkage which can form various motions. The most common linkages are one degree of freedom linkages in which one input motion generates one output motion. In planar linkages, the motions are formed in one plane.

The degrees of freedom or mobility of a planar linkage is calculated from the Kutzbach-Gruebler Eq. (4.6):

$$M = 3(n - 1) - 2f \tag{4.6}$$

where M is degrees of freedom, n is number of links including a single ground link, and f is number of one degree of freedom joints.

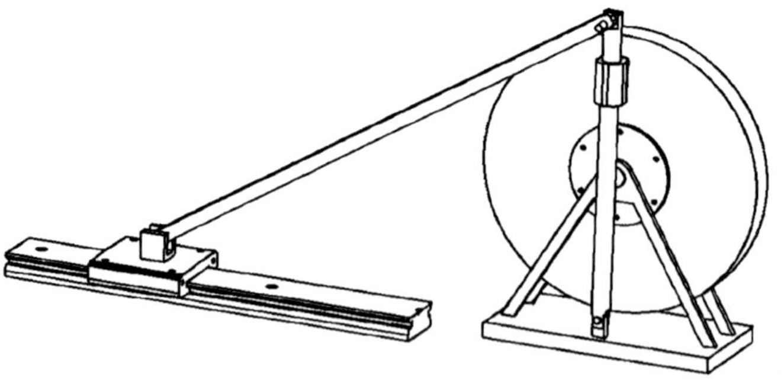

FIGURE 4.15 The linkage mechanism.

The most common joints are revolute joints, prismatic joints, and spherical or ball and socket joints. A revolute joint has one degree of freedom rotation and includes bearings, bolted joints, hinges, etc. A prismatic joint has one or two degrees of freedom linear motion and includes linear bearings, pistons, etc. A spherical or ball and socket joint has three degrees of freedom rotation.

4.7 Bearings

Bearings are used in applications in which a relative motion between two elements is required. Bearings can be generally classified into two groups, namely, sliding bearings or plain surface bearings (which have a thin layer or film of lubricant) and rolling bearings (which have a combination of rolling motion and lubrication).[5] Lubrication is required in most bearings to reduce friction between surfaces and remove generated heat.

Bearings are available in various types. Some common bearings are ball bearing, roller bearing, guide rails, and linear bearing. A ball bearing, shown in Fig. 4.16, is a type of rolling bearing which has balls to reduce rotational friction and support radial and axial loads. In a ball bearing, the load is transmitted from the outer race to the ball and from the ball to the inner race. The ball is spherical and contacts the inner and outer race at a very small point. Although this small contact area causes a smooth motion, when the ball bearing is overloaded, it may be ruined. An axial ball bearing used for the transmission of axial loads is shown in Fig. 4.17.

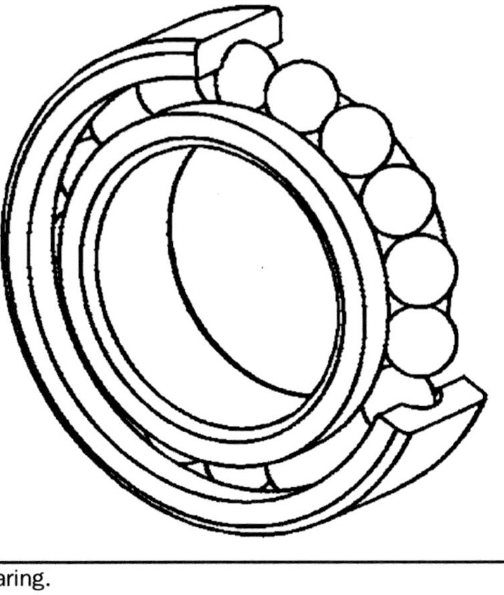

FIGURE 4.16 The ball bearing.

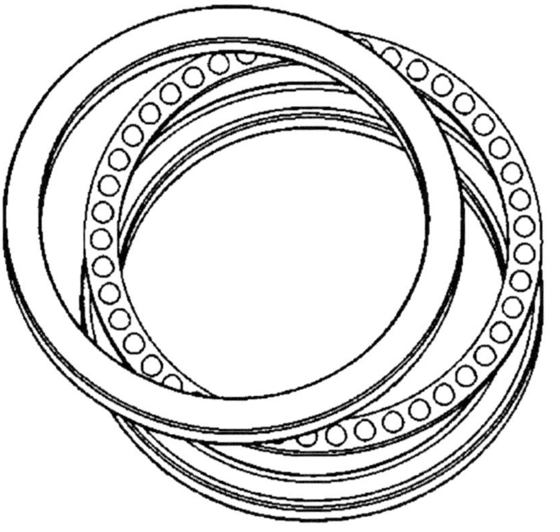

Figure 4.17 The axial bearing.

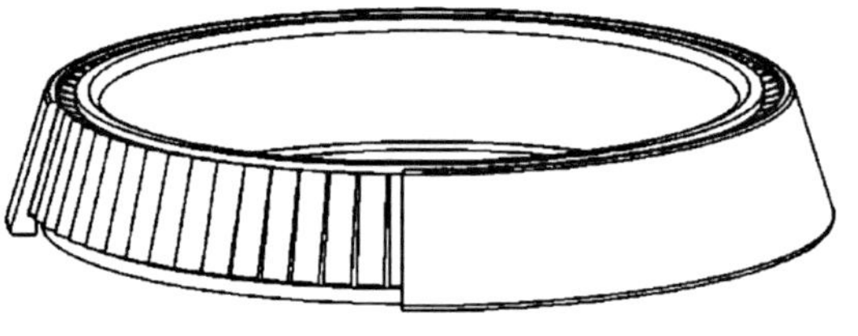

Figure 4.18 The roller bearing.

A roller bearing, shown in Fig. 4.18, has cylindrical rollers and the contact between the inner and outer race is in a line. Because the contact area is larger than that in ball bearings, the roller bearing can handle much greater loads.

A linear guide rail bearing, shown in Fig. 4.19, is used to provide accurate linear motion in one dimension.

A linear bearing, shown in Fig. 4.20, is also a bearing used to provide linear motion especially for short traveling distances.

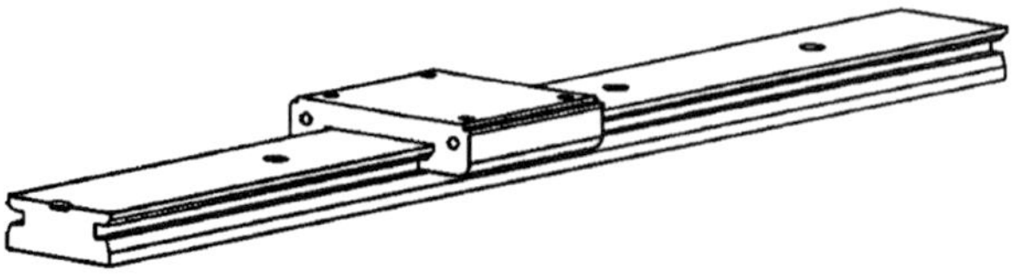

Figure 4.19 Linear guide rail.

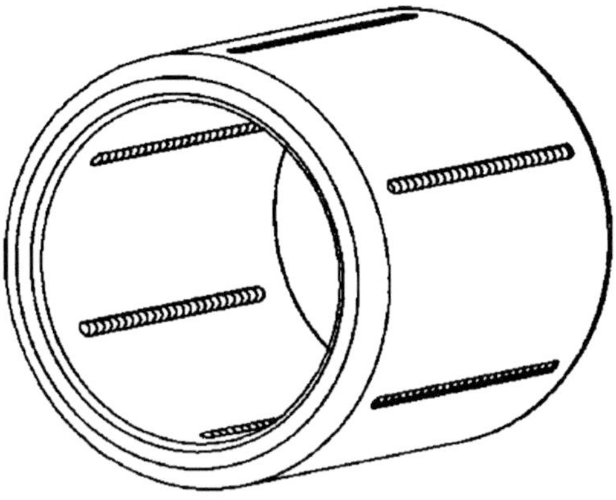

FIGURE 4.20 The linear bearing.

References

1. G. C. Onwubolu. *Mechatronics Principles and Applications*, Elsevier, 2005.
2. P. E. Sandin. *Robot Mechanisms and Mechanical Devices Illustrated*, McGraw-Hill, 2003.
3. Z. Li, W. W. Melek, and C. M. Clark. "Decentralized Robust Control of Robot Manipulators with Harmonic Drive Transmission and Application to Modular and Reconfigurable Serial Arms," *Robotica*, vol. 27, no. 2, 2009, pp. 291–302.
4. Timing Belt Theory, Gates Mectrol, 2006, www.gatesmectrol.com.
5. P. R. N. Childs. *Mechanical Design*, Elsevier, 2d ed., 2004.
6. V. B. Bhandari. *Design of Machine Elements*, 3d ed., Tata McGraw-Hill, 2010.

CHAPTER 5

Processing and Control Systems

5.1 Introduction

In previous chapters, an explanation was given on the purpose, fabrication, and function of sensors and transducers together with a range of mechanical systems and mechanisms. This chapter presents a description of the principles and methods of processing and controlling mechatronics systems and includes the basics of control, data acquisition, microprocessors, and microcontrollers.

5.2 Basics of Control

A control system is set of electronic devices and equipment which are in place to ensure stability, accuracy, and smooth transition of a process or any manufacturing activity.[1] The device or system to be controlled is called the plant or the process, and the component that controls it is called the controller. The system requires some form of excitation as an input and the behavior of the system is described according to its output.

Control systems can be either linear or nonlinear. A linear control system is one in which the superposition principle can be applied so, therefore, it must be both additive and homogeneous and it is these two properties that constitute the superposition principle. The additive property is expressed as shown in Eq. (5.1):

$$f(x+y) = f(x) + f(y) \tag{5.1}$$

where x and y belong in the domain of function f. The homogeneous property is expressed by Eq. (5.2):

$$f(ax) = af(x) \tag{5.2}$$

where x belongs in the domain of the function f and a is a scalar constant.

It is very difficult to design a linear system that satisfies the superposition principle perfectly because the phenomena inherent within most physical systems (such as friction forces, saturation, backlash, dead zone, etc. are, in themselves, nonlinear). Because it is both difficult and time consuming to solve nonlinear system problems, they are generally approximated with linear systems for a limited range of operation.

Control systems can be either time varying or time invariant. In a time varying control system, the parameters vary with time; in a time invariant system, the parameters are constant and do not vary with time during the operation of the system. The design and analysis of time varying control systems are, generally, much more complex than the design and analysis of time invariant control systems. Electrical networks, including elements such as resistances, inductances, and capacitances, are time invariant systems which have constant parameters that are not the function of time.[2] An important classification of control systems is open-loop and closed-loop systems. In an open-loop control system, the output is dependent on the input but has no effect on either the control action or the input itself. In an open-loop control system, the reference input is applied to the controller which sends an actuating signal to control the process. It follows, therefore, that since, in an open-looped system, the process itself generates the desired controlled output it is not, therefore, compared with the reference input. An open-loop control system is shown in Fig. 5.1.

Although open loop control systems have certain advantages, such as being simple to construct, economical, highly convenient (when the output is difficult to measure), consume less power and are generally more stable, they do also have some disadvantages. For instance, because there is no feedback to the controller, if the output device does not operate as instructed there is no way for the system to know. Also, occasional calibration is necessary in order to maintain its accuracy and reliability because they are dependent on the accurate precalibration of the controller. They are also unable to sense environmental changes and so tend to give inaccurate results under variations in ambience and are unable to sense internal disturbances in the system after the controller stage.[2,3] To overcome these disadvantages, closed-loop control systems are used in which the input, or the controlling action, is dependent upon the output. Closed-loop control systems use the useful properties of feedback to make decisions about variations in the control signal that actuates the plant. In a closed-loop control system, the output is fed back to the input to be compared with the reference input applied to it. The output signal of the feedback component is called the feedback signal and is compared with the reference input. The difference is the error signal of the system which is fed back to the controller to reduce it in order to produce the desired output. The error signal is modified by the controller and causes a response in the plant such that the error signal is continually being reduced to the point where it approaches zero. A closed-loop control system is shown in Fig. 5.2.

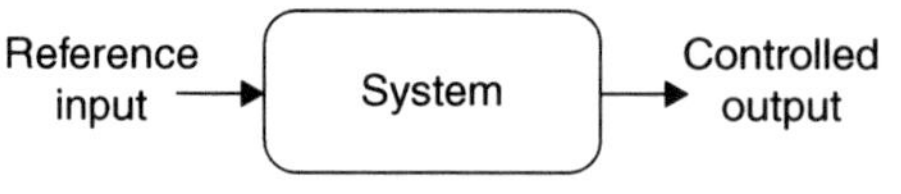

FIGURE 5.1 Open-loop control system.

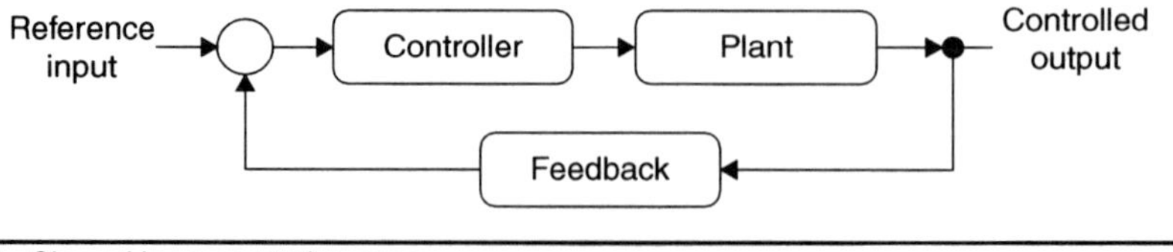

FIGURE 5.2 Closed-loop control system.

There are three techniques for closed-loop control systems, including proportional, derivative, and integral control techniques. Proportional control is a linear feedback in which the signal driving the motor or actuator is directly proportional to the difference between the input signal and the actual measured output. In integral control, the signal that drives the motor or actuator equals the time integral of the difference between the input signal and the actual measured output. In derivative control, the signal driving the motor, or actuator, is proportional to the time derivative of the difference between the input signal and the actual measured output. Although proportional control is the simplest form of feedback, the two other techniques are also required to compensate for steady-state errors that cannot be removed from proportional control.[4] Proportional-integral-derivative (PID) control is the combination of these three techniques in which the signal driving the motor or actuator equals the weighted sum of the difference, the time integral of the difference, and the time derivative of the difference between the input signal and the actual measured output.

Closed-loop systems have many advantages such as high accuracy and reliability because the controller modifies the actuating signal such that any error in the system will be reduced to zero. This system is also able to sense environmental changes, as well as internal disturbances, so it is able to modify the error. Additionally, it reduces the effect of nonlinearities and distortions, and operates at a very high frequency zone (bandwidth). The disadvantages, however, are that they consume more power, are more complex and expensive, generate spurious oscillations in the system caused as a result of attempting to correct any error. It is, therefore, these problems of instability that need to be considered when designing such a system.[2,3] When designing a control system, in the modeling procedure it is important to first define the system and its control objectives. The system is then modeled and a qualitative description of the system is translated into a functional block diagram that describes the various elements of the system in the form of a schematic diagram. After preparing the schematic diagram of the physical system, the physical laws, including the Kirchoff's laws for electrical systems (which deal with the conservation of charge and energy in an electrical circuit) and Newton's laws for mechanical systems (which deal with the relationship between the various forces acting on a body and its motion due to those forces), will be used and the assumptions will be simplified to model the system mathematically. The two common methods for the mathematical modeling of control systems are transfer function in the frequency domain and state space representation in the time domain.[5]

5.2.1 Modeling in the Frequency Domain

It is complicated to model a control system in the form of a block diagram when the system is described by differential equations. The Laplace transform is a very useful integral transform applicable in representing the input, output, and system, separately. The Laplace transform converts the differential equations of a system to a transfer function which is a term used to describe the mathematical function of parameters in a control system. A mathematical model is then obtained to relate the output of the system to the input in algebraic form.

Laplace transforms simplify the representation of physical systems and is defined as shown in Eq. (5.3):

$$L\left[f(t)\right] = F(s) = \int_0^{\infty} f(t)e^{-st}dt \tag{5.3}$$

where $s = \sigma + j\omega$ is a complex number. $F(s)$ is the Laplace transform which is calculated by knowing $f(t)$ and the integral in Eq. (5.3). The inverse Laplace transform is used to determine $f(t)$ by knowing $F(s)$ and is defined as shown in Eq. (5.4):

$$L^{-1}\left[F(s)\right] = \frac{1}{2\pi j}\lim_{\omega\to\infty}\int_{\sigma-j\omega}^{\sigma+j\omega} F(s)e^{st}ds = f(t)\,u(t) \tag{5.4}$$

where

$$u(t) = \begin{cases} 1 \text{ if } t \geq 0 \\ 0 \text{ if } t < 0 \end{cases}$$

is the unit step function.

The inverse Laplace transform of complicated functions can be determined by converting them into simpler functions which is known as the Laplace transform.

The transfer function relates the output of the control system to its input and permits division of the input, the output, and the system into three separate parts as shown in Fig. 5.3. The *Gain*, $G(s)$, is defined as the ratio of the output Laplace transform, $C(s)$, divided by the input Laplace transform, $R(s)$.

5.2.2 Modeling in the Time Domain

The time domain approach, or state space representation, is a method of mathematical modeling for physical systems in the form of input, output, and state variables related by first-order differential equations. This mathematical method is used for a wide range of systems including nonlinear time varying systems. The steps in state space representation are: selecting a special subset of possible variables called state variables, writing n simultaneous, first-order differential equations called state equations for an nth-order system in terms of the state variables, considering the initial condition of all the state variables; at t_0 as well as the system input for $t \geq t_0$, solving the simultaneous differential equations for the state variables for $t \geq t_0$, combining the state variables with the input of the system with an algebraic equation called the output equation and finding all of the other variables for $t \geq t_0$, considering the state equations and the output equations as a viable representation of the system called state space representation.[5]

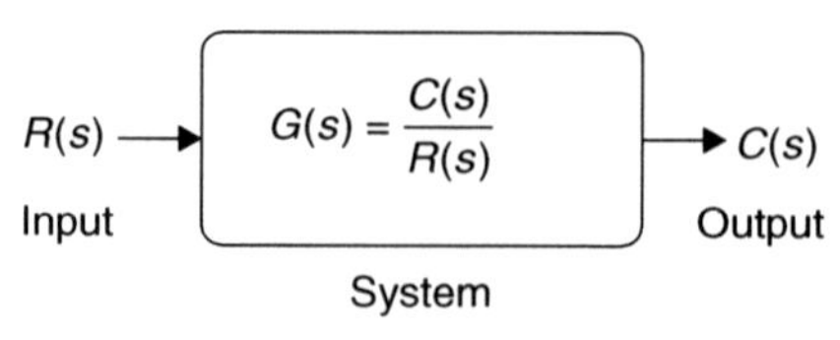

FIGURE 5.3 The block diagram of a transfer function.

A system is represented in state space by two equations. The state equation is shown in Eq. (5.5) and the output equation shown in Eq. (5.6), for $t \geq t_0$ and initial conditions, $x(t_0)$:

$$\dot{x} = Ax + Bu \tag{5.5}$$

$$y = Cx + Du \tag{5.6}$$

where x is the state vector; $\dot{x}$ is the derivative of the state vector with respect to time; y is the output vector; u is the input or control vector; A is the state matrix; B is the input matrix; C is the output matrix; and D is the feed forward matrix.

5.3 Data Acquisition

Data acquisition systems are used to acquire analog signals from the environment and convert them into digital form to process and record data. Analog signals acquired by data acquisition are mostly electrical output signals from sensors and transducers that measure physical quantities such as temperature, flow, pressure, stress or strain, etc. The flow of information in data acquisition systems is generally as follows.[5]

1. Input transducers measure some property of the environment.
2. Analog output from the transducers is then conditioned (amplified, filtered, etc.).
3. It is digitized using an analog to digital converter (ADC).
4. This information is then acquired, processed, and recorded by the computer.
5. The computer may then modify the environment by outputting control signals.
6. These are converted to analog signals using a digital-to-analog converter (DAC).
7. These signals are then conditioned (e.g., amplified and filtered) appropriately for an output transducer.
8. The output transducer interacts with the environment.

5.3.1 Sampling and Aliasing

Although analog functions cannot be analyzed by digital computers directly, they may, nonetheless, need to be sampled. An analog signal, $v(t)$, which is a continuous function of time, can be represented as a discrete time signal by using values of $v(t)$ at intervals of nT_s to form $v[n]$. T_s is the sampling period taken at regular intervals. In sampling, the sampling rate frequency f_s (which is the inverse of T_s) is specified more often than the sampling period and is measured in hertz. During high sampling rates, the points can simply be connected to each other by small linear lines and construct the signal $v(t)$ from $v[n]$, approaching the analog signal. The discrete samples are then digitized and processed by a computer. Figure 5.4*a* shows an analog signal and Fig. 5.4*b* shows its sampled form.

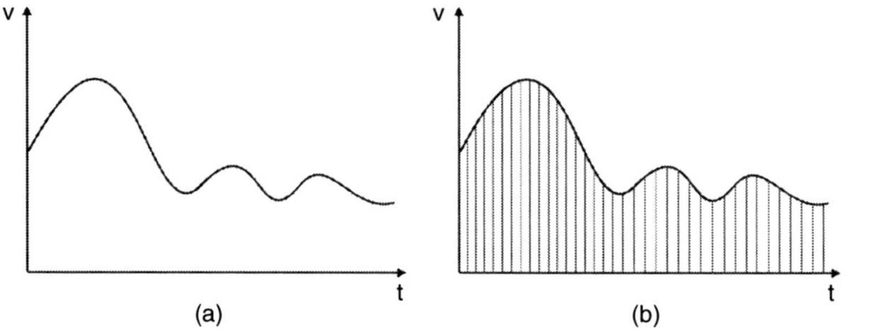

FIGURE 5.4 Digitizing a signal: (*a*) Analog signal, (*b*) sampled signal.

When the frequency of a signal is high, and the signal has significant variation, then the sampling period of the signal must be small enough to approximate the signal correctly which means that, for high frequency signals, a correspondingly high sample rate is required. A common distortion in digital processing applications is aliasing which occurs when the frequencies of the analog signal is larger than one half of the sampling rate. Removing aliasing is called anti-aliasing in which the analog signal is generally filtered by a low-pass filter before being sampled.

5.3.2 Quantization and Coding

When the signal is sampled, it must be quantized. Quantization is the process of mapping a large set of input values to a smaller set such as rounding values to some unit of precision which, in this case, is the process of transforming a continuous analog voltage into a discrete number of voltage states. Because digital computers operate using the binary system, the number of these possible states, N, is equal to the number of bit combinations, as shown in Eq. (5.7):

$$N = 2^n \tag{5.7}$$

where n is the number of quantization bits.

The quantized signal must then be digitally coded (transforming the quantized signals into a digital representation) during which each quantization state is given a unique label.

5.3.3 Analog-to-Digital Converter

The analog-to-digital converter (ADC) is used to convert an analog signal into a continuous digital signal that can then be fed into a computer for processing. The ADC is generally classified by two parameters: namely, the analog input range and the digital output range.[6] A block diagram of an ADC system contains the following six prerequisite elements.[5]

1. Sensor (which provides the analog signal to the system)
2. Buffer amplifier (that amplifies the sensor signal in a range close to, but not exceeding, the full input voltage range of the ADC)

3. Low-pass filter (used to remove undesirable high-frequency components in the signal that could generate aliasing)
4. Sample-and-hold amplifier (which maintains a fixed input value during the short conversion time)
5. Analog-to-digital converter
6. Computer

5.3.4 Digital-to-Analog Converter

A digital-to-analog converter (DAC) converts a digital signal into a continuous analog signal. Since the output command from the computer is in binary form, a digital-to-analog converter is required to convert the command into a digital signal and act as an interface between the computer and an output transducer. The smoothness of the signal representation depends upon the number of bits accepted by the digital-to-analog converter and the output range required.[6]

5.4 Microprocessors and Microcontrollers

Many mechatronics systems have multiple inputs and outputs within which complex relationships must be controlled. In such systems, hardware solutions are usually not practical so a microprocessor-based system using software is required. Software is a set of instructions used to perform logic and arithmetic functions and access input/output signals. It can be modified easily to change the system's functionality without the need to change any hardware.

A microprocessor is a very large scale integration (VLSI) programmable chip consisting of digital circuits that execute arithmetic, logic, communication, and control functions. A collection of these, in conjunction with a microprocessor and other components such as interface and memory chips, is called a microcomputer. This actually is a complete computer but on a much smaller scale.

The microprocessor performs all, or most, of the functions of a computer's central processing unit (CPU). It is contained on a single integrated circuit and is used to perform all primary computation and system control operations. The arithmetic logic unit (ALU) is located inside the CPU and executes mathematical functions on data structured as binary words.

The following terminology describes some useful terms in microcomputer systems:[5,7]

- A bit (short for binary *digit*), the smallest unit of information on a machine. A single bit can hold only one of two values: 0 or 1.
- A word is a set of bits, usually with a length of 8, 16, 32, or 64 bits.
- The instruction decoder is a part of microprocessor that decodes coded instructions which come from memory by the control unit and are stored in the instruction register. Each instruction commands the ALU to perform bit manipulation on words stored in the data registers. The ALU results are also stored in CPU data registers and are transferred to memory by the control unit.

- The bus is a collection of conductors that acts as the central nervous system of the computer. The bus consists of data, address, and control lines which permit a particular component to access data addressed to that component. Each component connected to the bus has its own bus controller. Data lines are two-way lines which carry data around the various system components. Address lines are one-way lines which transfer addresses from the microprocessor to the memory or other devices. Control lines are used to transport read and write signals, the system clock signal, and other control signals.
- The read only memory (ROM) is a permanent storage of data. Data on ROM can be read by the CPU, but the CPU cannot write data to it. ROM does not need any power supply to hold its data.
- Random access memory (RAM) stores data during the program run-time. Data can be read from or written to the RAM at any time. Data in the RAM is lost whenever the power is turned off.
- Erasable programmable read only memory (EPROM): Data stored in an EPROM can be erased and the EPROM can be rewritten many times. An EPROM can be erased electrically or with ultraviolet light applied through a transparent quartz window on top of the EPROM IC.
- Machine code is a set of binary code instructions that can be performed by the CPU. In/out (I/O) devices connected to the bus are used for communication to and from the microprocessor and external computer peripheral I/O devices include keyboards, displays, printers, modems, and network devices. In mechatronics applications, analog-to-digital (A/D), digital-to-analog (D/A), and digital-to-digital (D/D) I/O devices act as interfaces between the microcomputer, switches, sensors, and actuators.
- *Assembler* is a program used in microprocessors that converts assembly language into machine code which the microprocessor can understand. Programs can also be written in a higher level language such as BASIC or C, for which the microprocessor will need a compiler to understand.

Most of the recent advances in microprocessor technology have been in the realm of either CPUs or development of microcontrollers.[5] The microcontroller, which is essentially a microcomputer on a single IC, is small and can be physically embedded in mechatronics systems.

The components of a microcontroller are: the CPU, RAM, ROM, digital I/O ports, a serial communication interface, timers, analog-to-digital (A/D) converters, and digital-to-analog (D/A) converters.

The CPU controls all the components in a microcontroller. The RAM stores settings and values used when a program is being executed and the ROM stores permanent data. Programming devices can be used to download a compiled machine code file from a PC to the EEPROM (electrically erasable programmable ROM), via the PC serial port and special purpose pins on the microcontroller. Data in the EEPROM is nonvolatile so it is still is accessible even after the microcontroller power is off. The digital I/O ports transfer binary data to and from the microcontroller using external pins which can be used to read the state of switches and on/off sensors. Some common standards or protocols for serial communication are SPI (serial peripheral interface), I^2C (inter-integrated circuit),

UART (universal asynchronous receiver transmitter), and USART (universal synchronous asynchronous receiver transmitter).[5] As previously mentioned, the ADC converts an external analog voltage to a digital value and the DAC converts a digital voltage to an analog voltage that can be used by any non-digital device such as a motor amplifier. Microcontrollers, typically, have less program memory than microcomputers and their clock speeds are usually slower also.[5]

References

1. L. J. Nagrath and M. Gopal. *Control Systems Engineering*, 4th ed., New Age International Publishers, 2006.
2. S. C. Goyal and U. A. Bakshi. *Principles of control systems*, 7th ed., Technical Publication, 2008.
3. A. A. Kumar. *Control Systems*, PHI Learning, 2007.
4. P. E. Sandin. *Robot Mechanisms and Mechanical Devices Illustrated*, McGraw-Hill, USA, 2003.
5. G. C. Onwubolu. *Mechatronics Principles and Applications*, Elsevier, 2005.
6. R. H. Bishop (Ed.). *The Mechatronics Hand Book*, CRC Press, 2002.
7. J. Crisp. *Introduction to Microprocessors and Microcontrollers*, 2d ed., Elsevier/Newnes, 2004.

CHAPTER 6

Artificial Intelligence and Expert Systems

6.1 Introduction

Previous chapters have presented an introduction to mechatronics, the fundamentals of sensing technology, a description of actuators and feedback sensors, basic mechanisms, and mechanical devices followed by a description of processing and control systems. Currently, equipment and processes used in the industrial sector, as well as medical institutions, are growing in complexity that place imposing demands upon current control methods. The software employed in many systems today is required, more than ever, to replicate human intelligence and is used in advanced systems that speedily convert required data using advanced search engines.

Medical artificial intelligence is primarily concerned with the construction of artificial intelligence (AI) programs that perform diagnosis and make therapy recommendations. Unlike medical applications based on other programming methods, such as purely statistical and probabilistic methods, medical AI programs are based on symbolic models of disease entities and their relationship to patient factors and clinical manifestations. Much of the difficulty has been the poor way in which they have fitted into clinical practice, either solving problems that were not perceived to be an issue or imposing changes in the way clinicians worked. What is now being realized is that when they fill an appropriate role, intelligent programs do indeed offer significant benefits. One of the most important tasks now facing the developers of AI based systems is to characterize accurately those aspects of medical practice that are best suited to the introduction of AI systems.

The purpose of this chapter, therefore, is to discuss and extol the virtues of intelligent mechatronics systems in the field of medicine and biomedical engineering. It is not feasible to mention the various specifications and properties of all intelligent systems so only the most important ones are presented and, if more information is desired, the reader can check the relevant references. The main concepts discussed in this chapter are artificial intelligence, expert systems, artificial neural networks, fuzzy systems, and neuro fuzzy systems.

6.2 Artificial Intelligence

Artificial intelligence (AI), a term first coined John McCarthy in 1956, is a branch of computer science which focuses on the development of computer systems to simulate the processes of problem solving and to duplicate human brain functions and are used to solve problems inherent within complex systems. Hence, AI can be defined as being the methods used to solve complex problems based on the intelligent behavior of humans and other animate life-forms.[1]

There are various areas in AI, including artificial life, machine learning, computer vision, multi-agent systems, planning, and playing games. Much research in AI is performed in the field of cognitive psychology which studies mental processes, including how people think, perceive, remember, and learn. Cognitive psychology is not to be confused with behavioral psychology, also known as behaviorism, which is a theory of learning based upon the idea that all behaviors are acquired through conditioning caused by interaction with the environment.

6.2.1 Semantic Net

Semantic nets are two-dimensional representations of knowledge that can be defined as being labeled directed graphs. They consist of nodes, links (edges), and link labels. In the semantic network diagram, nodes appear as circles, ellipses, or rectangles to represent objects such as physical objects, concepts, or situations. Links appear as arrows to express the relationships between objects, and link labels specify particular relations. A good example of a semantic net is the diagram of a family tree in which nodes represent people, and edges represent parental relationships or relationships by marriage. Figure 6.1 shows a simple semantic net.

6.2.2 Semantic Tree

A semantic tree is a kind of semantic net, in which each node (except for the root node) has exactly one predecessor (parent) and one or more successors (children). A semantic net and a semantic tree are shown in Fig. 6.2. In the semantic tree in Fig. 6.2, node A is

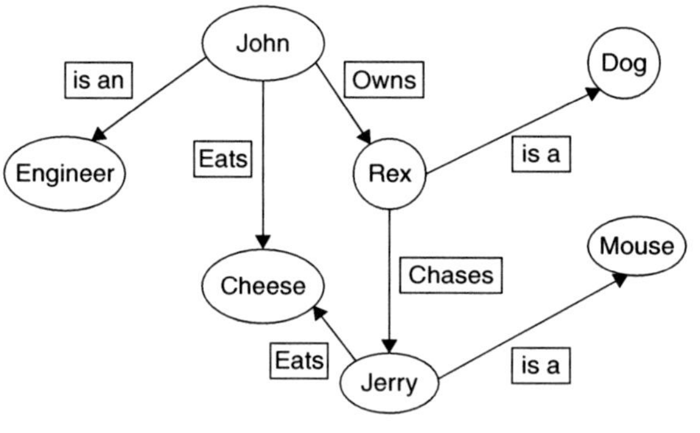

FIGURE 6.1 A simple semantic net.

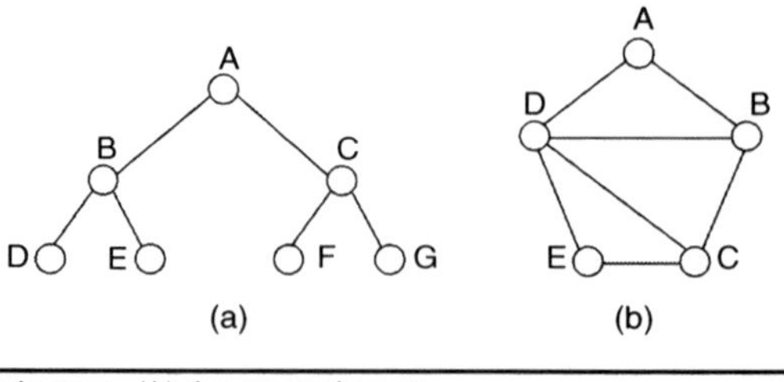

FIGURE 6.2 (*a*) A semantic tree. (*b*) A semantic net.

the predecessor of node B and node C, and connects by one edge to node B and node C. Node A comes before nodes B and C in the tree. The successors of node B are nodes D and E which are connected directly to node B and come after it in the tree.

The relationships of node B can be written as: succ (B) = D and pred (B) = A.

6.2.3 Combining Frames with Rules

Frames or semantic nets often have procedures that enable a system to act according to data within the frames. Frames can be combined with rules. A frame-based system with rules will use rules to draw conclusions, and when it cannot find a value for a particular slot, a WHEN-NEEDED procedure will run to find the required value.[1] If no value is found from that procedure, then the user will be asked to provide a value.

6.2.4 Search Spaces

A search space is a set of possible options in a problem, in which one or more of those options are the solution to that problem. For instance, when the meaning of a particular word is required in a dictionary, the search space includes all the pages of dictionary.

6.2.5 Combinatorial Explosion

In many problems, by increasing the number of items to be considered, the number of possible paths in the search space increases exponentially such that, in order to solve the problem, the processing time becomes greatly protracted.

6.2.6 Problem Reduction

This involves reducing the main aspects of a problem into smaller segments in which the solution to each of these entities will provide an ultimate resolution to the larger problem.

6.2.7 Forward Chaining and Backward Chaining Search

There are two main techniques for searching a search tree: forward chaining and backward chaining. Forward chaining starts with facts and searches forward through the rules to find a desired goal. Backward chaining starts with a goal and then searches back through inference rules to find the facts that support the goal. Of these two methods, the one to use is determined by the problem itself. A comparison of conditions to actions in the rule base can help determine which chaining method is preferred. If the average rule has more conditions than conclusions, forward chaining is favored. If the opposite holds true and the average rule is imbued with more conclusions than conditions such that each fact may fan out into a large number of new facts or actions, backward chaining is ideal. If neither is dominant, the number of facts in the working memory may help the decision. If all (relevant) facts are already known, and the purpose of the system is to find where that information leads, forward chaining should be selected. If, on the other hand, few or no facts are known and the goal is to find if one of many possible conclusions is true, backward chaining should be used.

6.2.8 Search Methods

The two most common search methods are depth-first search and breadth-first search. The depth-first search checks each path to its greatest depth before going to the next path. The breadth-first search traverses a search tree by breadth and starts at the root node and checks all neighboring nodes to find the goal. The depth-first search has much lower memory requirements and works well when the goal node is near the bottom of the tree. The breadth-first search is ideal in situations where the answer is close to the top of the tree.

6.2.9 Properties of Search Methods

Search methods have various properties, including complexity, completeness, optimality, and irrevocability.[1]

Complexity embraces both the amount of time needed to complete the search in conjunction with the amount of space required to accomplish this goal.

Completeness is the assuredness that if the stated goal does indeed exist for a problem, it will eventually be found.

Optimality is achieving the stated goal by using the least number of actions.

Irrevocability does not use backtracking and examines just one path. This method is also described as being tentative, an example of which is a depth-first search.

6.2.10 Logic

Theoretical computer science developed out of logic and some related areas of mathematics. So theoretically minded computer scientists are well informed about logic even when they are not logicians. Computer scientists, in general, are familiar with the idea that logic provides techniques for analyzing the inferential properties of languages and with the distinction between a high-level logical analysis of a reasoning problem and its implementations. Logic, for instance, can provide a specification for a programming language by characterizing a mapping from programs to the computations that they license. A compiler that implements the language can be incomplete, or even unsound, as long as in some sense it only approximates the logical specification. This makes it possible for the involvement of logic in AI applications to vary from relatively weak uses in which the logic informs the implementation process with analytic insights, to strong uses in which the implementation algorithm can be shown to be sound and complete. In some cases, a working system is inspired by ideas from logic, but acquires features that at first seem logically problematic but can later be explained by developing new ideas in logical theory.

In this regard, logic is used as a representational method for AI. Logic language can be used in systems that can understand and analyze human language. In classical logic, it is not possible to reason about possibilities. However, in some versions of logic such as probabilistic methods and fuzzy logic, it is possible to reason in uncertain situations.[1]

6.2.11 Playing Games

One of the most interesting areas of AI research has been in playing games. In 1997, the chess playing computer Deep Blue defeated the (then) reigning world chess champion, Garry Kasparov, in a six-game match. Although Deep Blue was a mainframe computer, far more powerful than the average home computer at that time, PCs have come a long way since then and chess programs are now available that can easily beat the vast majority of human players.

The structure of the software in these games is based on tree structures similar to (but vastly more complicated than) the semantic trees referred to previously in this chapter.

6.3 Expert Systems

An expert system is a computer application that solves complicated problems that would otherwise require extensive human expertise. In order to accomplish this, it simulates the human reasoning process by applying specific knowledge and interfaces. Expert systems also use human knowledge to solve problems that normally would require human intelligence. These expert systems represent expertise knowledge as data or rules within the computer which can be called upon when needing to solve problems. Books and manual guides have a tremendous amount of knowledge, but a human has to read and interpret the knowledge for it to be used. The first expert systems appeared in the late sixties as an adjunct to AI and, today, they exist in many forms, from medical diagnosis to investment analysis, from counseling to production control. Due to the advances of the last decade, today's expert systems users can choose from dozens of commercial software packages. At present, we accept as routine, such expert systems as weather forecasting, online mapping and driving directions, diagnostic systems for automotive repair shops, and so on. However, applications that are computational or deterministic in nature are not good options for this system because of the fact that it lacks common sense and is unable to make creative responses under unusual circumstances.[2]

6.3.1 Expert Systems Structure

An expert system generally consists of three main parts: knowledge base, working memory, and an inference engine. The knowledge base constitutes the problem-solving rules, facts, or intuition that a human expert might use in solving problems in a given problem domain and is usually stored in terms of if/then rules. It contains highly specialized knowledge on the particular problem area as provided by the expert in the form of statistical analysis, empirical or semiempirical rules, theoretical and computer simulation studies, and experimental testing.

The working memory represents relevant data for the current problem being solved and refers to task-specific data for the problem under consideration.

The inference engine is the control mechanism that organizes the problem data and searches through the knowledge base for applicable rules.[3]

6.3.2 Benefits of Expert Systems

Expert systems have various benefits, including the fact that they:[2]

- Increase the probability, frequency, and consistency of making good decisions.
- Facilitate real-time, low-cost expert decisions by a nonexpert.
- Increase the utilization of most of the available data.
- Help distribute human expertise.
- Allow objectivity by weighing evidence without bias and without regard for the user's personal and emotional reactions.
- Free the mind and time of the human expert to enable personal focusing on more creative activities.
- Encourage investigations into the complicated areas of a problem.
- Combine the knowledge of many experts in a specific field.

- Store an unlimited amount of information and work much faster than a human.
- Are available 24 hours a day, and be used from a distance via a network.

6.3.3 Heuristic Reasoning

The problem-solving method used by humans is called heuristic reasoning in which an expert is able to find a good solution quickly and efficiently. Conventional programs only recognize numeric or alphabetic strings and manipulate them in a preprogrammed manner, but expert systems use symbolic manipulation and heuristic inference processes which match the human thought process.[2]

6.4 Artificial Neural Network

Artificial neural networks (ANN) are composed of simple processing elements, capable of processing information in response to an external input. The physiology of the brain and the electronic processing part of computers are similar in that both manipulate large amounts of data. In computers, the basic unit of processing is the bit which is in either an on or off state. In the brain, data processing units are called neurons and work according to a binary principle of being in either an on or off state. When a neuron is on, it fires a signal to other neurons across a network of synapses and, when it is off, there is no firing. Neurons do not physically touch each other. The spaces between the transmitters of one and the antennae of another are called synapses, and it is these synaptic connections that are continually being made and unmade that form a vast, ever-changing neural network. While the physical alignment of neural cells is presently seen as being determined genetically, the synaptic connections between cells are malleable and constantly changing.

6.4.1 Neuron and Neurode

A biological nerve cell is composed of a cell body and a large number of branches called dendrites that collect sensory inputs to the cell body and assume the form of treelike extensions. Most neurons consist of multiple dendrites, which are short and typically highly branched. The specialty of dendrites is that they receive information and form synaptic contacts with the terminals of other nerve cells to allow nerve impulses to be transmitted. The dendrites themselves make contact with other nerve cells through a synapse and, when a nerve cell is activated, it fires an electrical signal which is sent along a conduit called an axon. When the electrical signal passes through a synapse, a number of chemical reactions are activated, causing specific chemicals to be released and collected by the dendrites which then fire when the receiving nerve cell has collected enough sensory inputs. A biological neuron is shown in Fig. 6.3.

A neurode, shown in Fig. 6.4, is an artificial neuron that simulates the biological model of a neural network and is supplied with several input signals and propagates one output signal.

Artificial neurons are arranged into layers in which the neurons from one layer are connected to the neurons in the two layers on either side. Figure 6.5 shows the basic structure of neural networks.

The network is arranged in such a way that the input layer receives inputs that are fed into each neuron in the next layer until it reaches the outer layer. The hidden layers are merely avenues of propagation and are not connected to the external world.

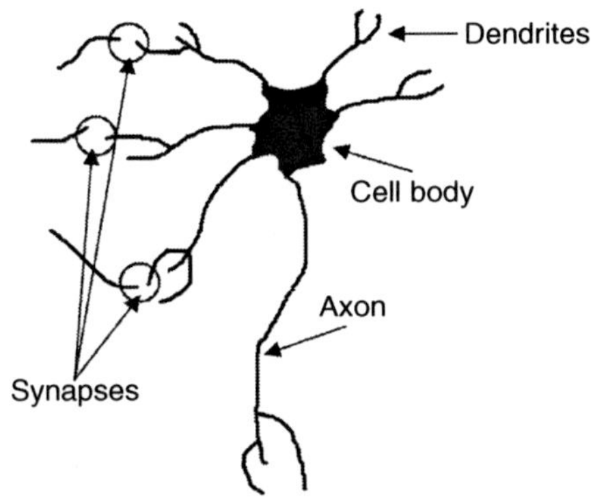

FIGURE 6.3 The biological neuron.

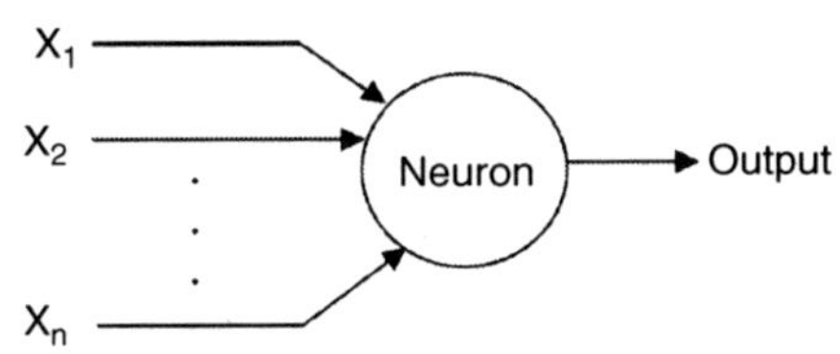

FIGURE 6.4 A neurode.

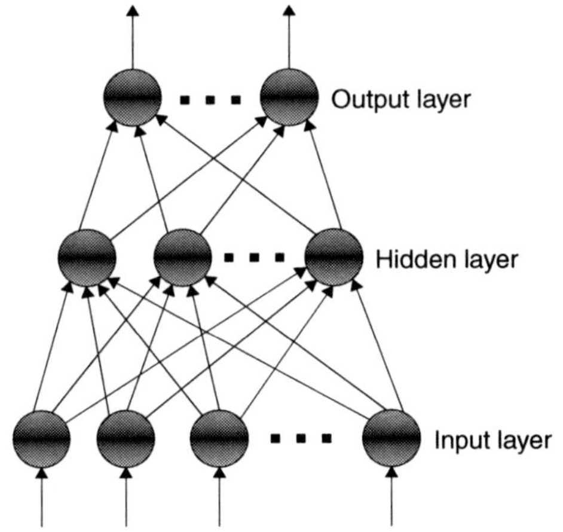

FIGURE 6.5 Neural network layers.

The connections between neurons are weighted (data is manipulated and calculated) and, by modifying these weighted factors, extremely complex classifications such as handwriting analysis and face recognition can be performed by the neural network.

Each synapse of a biological neuron represents an input of the neurode. The effectiveness of the synaptic junction is described by a multiplicative weight of that neurode input. The coincidence of the synaptic stimulation is modeled by a simple summation. The activation of the neurode is also defined by an activation of the weighted sum of the neurode input. The output o of a neurode can be expressed as shown in Eqs. (6.1) and (6.2):

$$o = f(\text{net}) \tag{6.1}$$

$$net = \sum_{i=1}^{N} w_i x_i \tag{6.2}$$

where x_i are the inputs, w_i are the weights associated with the inputs, and f is a nonlinear function. There are a total of N inputs. The same equation can also be expressed in matrix form as shown in Eq. (6.3):

$$o = f(W^T X) \tag{6.3}$$

where $W = [w_0, w_1, \ldots, w_N]$ and $X = [1, x_1, \ldots, x_N]$. Note that the constant threshold has been defined as x_0 and is set to 1.

The above definition emphasizes the similarities between the neurode and a linear combiner. A neurode, compared to a linear combiner, has an additional nonlinear transformation f. This transformation is often nonlinear. In cases that the transformation is a linear function, the neurode is the same as a linear combiner.[2]

6.4.2 Neural Network Learning

As discussed above, the neural network is a collection of simple, interconnected neurons. The neurons operate in parallel and store knowledge on the strength of connections between individual neurons. Such a parallel computing network can be used in intelligent tasks such as learning, speech synthesis, and pattern recognition.[3]

Artificial neural networks are based on some form of learning models and learn by evaluating changes in input data. Learning can be classified into supervised and unsupervised. In supervised learning, the network user assembles a set of training data which contains examples of inputs together with the corresponding outputs, and the network learns to infer the relationship between the two. Training data is usually taken from historical records. In unsupervised learning, there is no human intervention and input parameters are evaluated independently and recorded as patterns. The system evaluates various patterns and recognizes their similarities and dissimilarities. Unsupervised learning studies how systems can learn to represent particular input patterns in a way that reflects the statistical structure of the overall collection of input patterns.

6.4.3 Neural Network Training

Training a neural network includes the process of discovering the set of interconnection weights which causes a network output that satisfies a predefined criterion. In a supervised training method, feed forward neural networks are trained using the back propagation algorithm. In this method, the network has sample inputs and ideal responses, called a training pattern. The network is then trained to reproduce the ideal responses. Neural networks have capabilities of memorization, association, error tolerance, self-adaptation, and multiple complex pattern processing.[3] However, neural networks cannot explain their own reasoning behavior and cannot diagnose new phenomena.[3]

6.4.4 Neural Network Applications in Medicine

Medicine has always benefited from the forefront of technology. Technological advances in computers, lasers, ultrasonic imaging, etc., have boosted medicinal practice to extraordinary levels of achievement. ANN is currently the next promising area of interest. It is believed that neural networks will have extensive application to biomedical problems in the next few years. Already, it has been successfully applied to various areas of medicine such as diagnostic systems, biochemical analysis, image analysis, and drug development. Neural networks can be used in various fields of medicine, especially for diagnosis. Some of the common applications of neural network in medicine are presented as follows:[4]

Cardiology: Neural networks are used experimentally to model the human cardiovascular system. Diagnosis can be achieved by building a model of the cardiovascular system of an individual and comparing it with the real-time physiological measurements taken from the patient. If this routine is carried out regularly, potential harmful medical conditions can be detected at an early stage and thus the process of combating the disease can be made much easier.

Neurology: When attempting to make a diagnosis, it is sometimes difficult to differentiate between Alzheimer's disease and vascular dementia. A neural network analysis of brain single photon emission computed tomographic (SPECT) image data can be useful in these cases.

Gastroenterology: The prognosis for patients, upon whom a hepatectomy has been performed, must be given by medical personnel who are familiar with the overlapping fields of gastroenterology and oncology. A back propagation neural network has been prepared for this application.

Radiology: One of the most interesting and powerful applications of neural networks is in the field of radiology. In radiology, images that are acquired during the course of an examination contain a great deal of information, and hence are difficult to interpret using conventional rule-based systems. However, noise filtering and recognition of unusual images are easily accomplished through the auspices of neural network modeling due the esoteric prerogatives with which it is conferred.

EEG analysis: Because it is able to differentiate between physiological and pathological alterations, a number of neurological disorders can be examined by electroencephalogram (EEG) analysis. As in radiology, certain attributes of the neural network application, such as its flexibility and excellent adaptation capability, are useful in recognizing and processing the complex and diverse data obtained from an EEG examination.

Cytology: One of the most common applications of neural networks in medicine is the PAPNET system which uses neural net computer technology to analyze the conventional Pap smears. Neural network-based screening (NNS) of cervical smears can also be performed. It is now possible, however, for cytological diagnosis to be based on digital images generated by the NNS system although, for the sake of prudence, a so-called "hybrid screening method" is conducted in conjunction in which parts of these smears are additionally studied by microscope.

6.5 Fuzzy Systems

Fuzzy systems are used to represent concepts, ideas, and propositions. Fuzzy logic is a form of many-valued logic whose variables have a truth value that ranges in degree between 0 and 1. But in crisp logic, binary sets have two-valued logic which are only a 0 or 1. Fuzzy logic has been applied to many fields, from control theory to AI.

An approach to manage the uncertainty is the concept of fuzzy sets which was first introduced by Zadeh in 1965.[5] While neural networks are appropriate for modeling unknown systems and solving optimization problems, fuzzy systems represent problems and processing information and while there are many computational algorithms for processing numerical data, fuzzy systems manipulate information, not just data.[2]

In neural networks, AI is used that attempts to imitate the way a human brain works. Rather than using a digital model, in which all computations manipulate 0s and 1s, a neural network works by creating connections between processing elements, which is the computer equivalent of neurons and in which the organization and weights of the connections determine the output. In fuzzy logic, however, knowledge is stored in terms of rules and linguistic variables in which fuzzy inputs are processed to generate an acceptable response. Finally, the basic structure of the system is modeled.

6.5.1 Crisp Logic versus Fuzzy Logic

In classical set theory (crisp logic), a set consists of a collection of objects. Participation in the set is all or nothing. That is, an object is either a part of the set or it is not. Hence the characteristic function maps an element into either 0 (not in the set) or 1 (in the set).

However, in fuzzy set theory, the participation of an element in a set changes from all to nothing. In real life, there are many situations where the participation of an element in a set is not all or nothing. For example, a tall person is generally accepted to be someone whose height is more than 6 ft. When some persons whose height ranges from 5 to 7 ft are lined up, those toward the 7 ft end are considered to be tall, while those toward the 5 ft end are considered to be not tall. In fuzzy logic, whether or not the person is considered to be tall is a matter of degree whereas in crisp logic they are either tall or short depending upon the threshold. In the above example, this threshold is 6 ft and all the people under this height can be considered tall until a person joins the set who is more than 6 ft in height whereupon this person is considered to be tall and the others short. Fuzzy logic is a powerful problem-solving methodology with wide-ranging applications in industrial control and information processing. It provides a simple way to draw definite conclusions from vague, ambiguous, or imprecise information. It resembles human decision making by virtue of its ability to work from approximate data and find precise solutions. Unlike classical logic, which requires a deep understanding of a system, exact equations and precise numeric values, fuzzy logic incorporates an alternative way of thinking which allows modeling complex systems using a higher level of abstraction originating from our knowledge and experience. Fuzzy logic allows expressing this knowledge with subjective concepts such as "very good" and "a little bit satisfied" which are mapped into exact numeric ranges. It is, therefore, an appropriate technique for dealing with sources of inaccuracy and uncertainty that are nonstatistical in nature. A multivalued membership function is used in fuzzy logic to mark membership of an object in a class rather than the classical binary true or false values.

6.6 Neuro Fuzzy Systems

Neuro fuzzy is a field of AI that refers to combinations of ANN and fuzzy logic. Neuro fuzzy systems include the reasoning style of fuzzy systems and a linguistic model composed of a set of if/then fuzzy rules. Neuro fuzzy is a field of AI which consists of readable if/then statements that are almost a natural language, but it cannot learn the rules itself. The principles and development of ANN and fuzzy logic have advanced greatly in the past two decades. Neuro fuzzy systems are a multilayer feed forward adaptive networks that accomplish the basic elements and functions of conventional fuzzy logic systems.[6] Neuro fuzzy systems are used for modeling and controlling various complex systems, the most common of which being the adaptive network-based fuzzy inference system (ANFIS) developed by Jang,[7] fuzzy adaptive learning control network (FALCON) developed by Lin and Lee,[8] neuro-fuzzy control (NEFCON) proposed by Nauck, et al.,[9] generalized approximate reasoning-based intelligent control (GARIC) developed by Berenji and Khedkar,[10] and other variations from these developments.[11,12] These neuro fuzzy structures and systems laid the foundation stone of neuro fuzzy computing, and most conventional neuro fuzzy systems were developed on this original premise in which even more advanced features and methods are being adapted into the ever-growing sphere of applications and requirements.[6]

6.6.1 Neurons Performing Fuzzy Operations

A hybrid neuron is also a neuron with crisp inputs and crisp outputs. However, instead of performing a weighted (data manipulated and calculated) sum followed by a nonlinear transformation, a fuzzy neuron performs one of the fuzzy operations such as the triangular-norm or triangular-conorm operation. While this adaption of a neuron may not be based on proper biological concepts, the topology and architecture certainly are. A hybrid neuron has both crisp inputs and weights although, in general, arithmetic operations such as multiplication and addition are not used in combining inputs and weights because these functions tend to produce resultant values that do not necessarily lie in the interval between 0 and 1. Instead, fuzzy operations are preferred so that the resultant values do lie between the values of 0 and 1. Each input, and its corresponding weight, can be combined using a continuous operation such as t-norm or t-conorm. The aggregation of all weighted inputs can also be performed with any of the fuzzy continuous operations. If a nonlinear transformation is required, a continuous function, mapping the aggregation value to the output is used. One of the simplest types of hybrid systems is training a neural network to perform fuzzy logic functions. The main advantage of this method is the reduction of time complexity. There are many available neural network chips which can perform billions of neural connections in a second. If a neural network can be engineered to perform fuzzy operations, then the fuzzy operations can also be performed at the same speed.[2]

The three basic operations in classical set theory are: AND, OR, and NOT operations. The corresponding operations in fuzzy logic are min, max, and complement. When a fuzzy variable operates only between the values of 0 and 1, fuzzy operations work as a classical set. The terms conjunctive, disjunctive, and complement are used in more general settings to describe intersection, union, and complement operations.[2]

6.6.2 Regular Neural Network with Fuzzy Input and Output

In some problems, the input is a fuzzy value defined by the associated membership functions. A regular neural network can still be used in such problems. For solving such problems, one approach is to sample the membership function with a discrete number of domain values instead of working with a continuous interval.[2] So a set of membership values at discrete locations of the input parameter is the input of the neural network.

References

1. B. Coppin. *Artificial Intelligence Illuminated*, Jones and Bartlett Publishers, Inc., 2004.
2. B. Badiru and J. Y. Cheung. *Fuzzy Engineering Expert Systems with Neural Network Applications*, John Wiley and Sons, Inc., 2002.
3. R. H. Bishop (Ed.). *The Mechatronics Handbook*, CRC Press, 2002.
4. K. Papik, B. Molnar, R. Schaefer, Z. Dombovari, Z. Tulassay, and J. Feher. "Application of Neural Networks in Medicine—A Review," *Diagnostics and Medical Technology*, vol. 4, no. 3, 1998, pp. 538–546.
5. L. A. Zadeh. "*Fuzzy Sets, Information and Control*," vol. 8, 1965, pp. 338–353.
6. H. Li, C. L. Philip Ghen, and H. P. Huang. *Fuzzy Neural Intelligent Systems Mathematical Foundation and the Applications in Engineering*, CRC Press LLC, 2001.
7. J. S. Jang. "ANFIS: Adaptive-Network-Based Fuzzy Inference System," *IEEE Transactions on Systems, Man, and Cybernetics*, vol. 23, no. 3, 1993, pp. 665–684.
8. C. T. Lin and C. S. G. Lee. "Neural-network-based Fuzzy Logic Control and Decision System," IEEE Transactions on Computers, vol. 40, no. 12, 1991, pp. 1320–1336.
9. D. Nauck, F. Klawonn, and R. Kruse. *Foundations of Neuro-Fuzzy Systems*, Wiley, 1997.
10. H. R. Berenji and P. Khedkar, "Learning and Tuning Fuzzy Logic Controllers Through Reinforcements," *IEEE Transactions on Neural Networks*, vol. 3, no. 5, 1992, pp. 724–740.
11. C. T. Lin and C. S. G. Lee. *Neural Fuzzy Systems*, Prentice-Hall, 1996.
12. J. S. Jang, C. T. Sun, and E. Mizutani. *Neuro-Fuzzy and Soft Computing*, Prentice-Hall, 1997.

CHAPTER 7

Medical Imaging

7.1 Introduction

Medical imaging is undertaken to screen patients at risk for a disease, reduce uncertainty about a diagnosis in order to reassure patients and caregivers, assist with decisions about care choices, assess treatments and prognoses and/or guide surgery or other interventions. Medical images are the sources of valuable data with which a specialist can detect any abnormalities such as fractures, tumorous tissues, and stenosis in arteries. Nowadays, the majority of high-tech medical devices utilize digital technology and therefore can be embraced into mechatronics systems which, as stated in Chap. 1, are defined as being "the synergistic integration of mechanical engineering, with electronics and intelligent computer control in the design and manufacturing of industrial products and processes."

7.2 Medical Imaging Applications

In Fig. 7.1, a schematic representation of medical imaging in a mechatronics system is shown. For example, during the robotic biopsy of a tumorous tissue, the robot is steered and controlled by data provided by Magnetic Resonance Imaging (MRI). In this regard, and throughout this chapter, the general basis and function of different medical imaging systems, including ultrasound, MRI, CT scan and nuclear imaging are discussed.

7.2.1 Ultrasound

Ultrasound imaging, also called ultrasound scanning or sonography, involves exposing part of the body to high-frequency sound waves to produce pictures of the inside of the body and does not use ionizing radiation (as used in x-rays). Because ultrasound images are captured in real-time, they show the structure and movement of the body's internal organs, as well as blood flowing through blood vessels. Furthermore, ultrasound imaging is a noninvasive medical test that helps physicians diagnose and treat a large variety of medical conditions.[1]

In an ultrasound examination, a transducer sends the sound waves and records the echoing waves. When the transducer is pressed against the skin, it directs small pulses of inaudible, high-frequency sound waves into the body. As the sound waves bounce off internal organs, fluids and tissues, the sensitive microphone in the transducer records tiny changes in the sound's pitch and direction. These signature waves are instantly measured and displayed by a computer which, in turn, creates a real-time

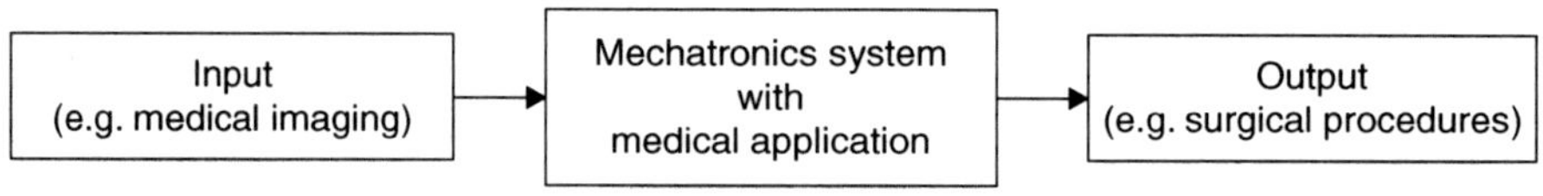

FIGURE 7.1 Schematic representation of medical imaging applications in a mechatronics system.

picture on a monitor. One or more frames of the moving pictures are typically captured as still images.

Since the introduction of ultrasound imaging systems, its probes have developed considerably. The first ultrasound probes consisted of a single element that was moved manually. Mechanical probes, which moved by means of a motorized device, were also introduced but it was considered that they lacked both agility and reliability.[2] There are three main types of transducers: linear, curved, and sector. The linear transducer is used primarily for small parts requiring high resolution and typically involves shallow depths. To achieve high resolution, higher frequencies are required. Since the elements are arranged in a linear fashion, the resulting image is rectangular. To broaden the field of view, a sector transducer is used. These transducers have a small footprint and are good for cardio applications due to small rib spacing. For abdominal viewing, curved transducers are typically used because of their geometrical, resolution, and penetration benefits.

The type of probe to use depends upon accessibility, the tissue being imaged, and the nature of the structures.[2] For example, if it is required to scan large structures (such as a fetal head) from a small aperture, a curved or phased array probe might be used. In contrast, when access is not an issue but a large imaging area near the probe is required (such as for carotid artery imaging), linear probes would be used.[2] In modern ultrasound systems, transducer elements are steered and focused by electronic beam formation, which can be divided into the simultaneous operations of focusing and steering.[3]

In focusing, the ultrasound system focuses sound waves along a given scan line so that the waves constructively add together in less than 5 μs at the desired focal point.[3] As the sound waves head toward the focal point, they reflect off on any object they encounter along their propagation path. Once all of the reflected waves have been measured with the transducers, new sound waves are transmitted toward a new focal point along the given scan line. Once all of the sound waves along the given scan line have been measured, the ultrasound system focuses along a new scan line until all of the scan lines in the desired region of interest have been measured.

Steering, also referred to as beam steering, is a method of steering the main lobe of a transducer to a certain direction. Array transducers have the ability to be steered as well as focused. Just as in focusing, the beam is directed by sequentially stimulating each element. This feature creates the sector scan by rapidly steering the beam from left to right in a matter of 15 μs to produce a 2D cross-sectional image.[3] Translation of the aperture is completed by switching in different groups of transducer elements to complete a linear scan of the active beam across the face of the array.

Image Quality Performance Parameters

There are four different parameters that could directly affect the quality of ultrasound images, namely, reflection, absorption, resolution, and dynamic range.[2]

Reflection Reflection of the sound beam occurs when it hits a boundary between materials having different acoustic impedance. The reflection (echo) is that portion of a sound wave that is returned from the boundary. The reflection time (the time taken for the wave to return to the probe) can be used to determine the depth of the object. The reflection within the body produces the ultrasound image, but should be minimized at an ultrasound couplant to the skin boundary where the couplant acts as an acoustic window through which the image is seen. The amount of sound waves which are reflected back at the interface between two tissues, is dependent upon the angle of incidence and the difference between the acoustic impedance values of the two tissues. If the difference is great, a large part of the sound waves will be reflected back. If too much sound is reflected back, and not enough waves remain to penetrate the tissue, the imaging will be poor. If, however, the difference is not great, a small amount will be reflected back to continue with ultrasound imaging. If the ultrasound beam meets a rough surface or small object, the beam is scattered in all directions and only a small amount will be received by the probe. For example, imaging the heart is particularly challenging since much of the acoustic window of the heart is hidden by the rib cage or the lungs. The contacting area between the transducer and the body sound might also be a problem since the sound waves could be strongly reflected at the transition plane. That is why a special acoustic gel is typically used to ensure that a good acoustic coupling is maintained between the transducer probe face and the body.[2]

Absorption Absorption is a parameter that changes with the type and depth of the tissue, and the attenuation and frequency of the sound. The absorbed dose is the ultrasonic power absorbed per unit of mass of an object, and is measured in watts per kilogram (W/kg) and increases with ultrasound intensity and frequency. The symbol for absorption is α, which is measured in dB/cm/MHz that can vary from 0.5 for fat to 2.0 for muscle.[4] Round-trip attenuation is given by 2α so, for typical tissue (fat), it is approximately 1 dB/cm/MHz.[2] For example, imaging at a depth of 5 cm at 2 MHz yields a round-trip attenuation of 10 dB, whereas imaging at a depth of 20 cm yields round-trip attenuation of 40 dB.

Resolution Resolution, or spatial resolution, in ultrasound imaging is a factor determined by three interacting effects.[5] Axial (or range or longitudinal) resolution is defined as the resolution along the direction of travel of the transmitted ultrasound beam and is limited by the length of the transmitted ultrasound pulse.[2] Elevational and azimuthal resolutions are two other factors that are determined by how well the ultrasound beam can be focused in these two orthogonal directions.[2] Another factor that is used when there is no difference between elevational and azimuthal focus is circular apertures such as annular arrays, which are composed of concentric ring transducers.[6]

Dynamic Range The dynamic range of an ultrasound signal is defined as being the maximum transmit pressure and the minimum detectable return signal. As discussed earlier, the transmit pressure is directly related to the required pulsing voltage. The maximum transmit pressure is strictly regulated by the FDA in the United States to reduce the chances of adverse events such as heating of tissue and mechanical bio effects such as cavitation.[7] The minimum receive voltage is completely technology dependent since it is currently limited by different noises such as that in the front-end preamplifier. However, assuming that this noise can be reduced, the noise in the sensor itself and the noise as a result of Brownian motion in the body will then set the minimum detectable signal.[4] Considering these factors, the total round-trip signal dynamic range is typically in the order of 120 dB for today's products.[2]

One of the main advantages of ultrasound imaging is its real-time aspect and its reasonable gray scale contrast of soft tissue structures.[8] Furthermore, these scanners are economical and are now also portable so they can be used by qualified personnel in any location. Another important positive property of ultrasound systems is that there are no known harmful effects of repeated ultrasound examinations, provided that the guidelines for the setting of the ultrasound emitted energy is followed.[8] One disadvantage, however, is its relatively poor spatial image resolution as a result of noise in most applications. Also, because its sound waves are mostly reflected from bones, a relatively large number of soft tissues cannot be imaged routinely.[8] Air in the lungs and thick fat layers also represent major problems for ultrasound imaging.

3D-ultrasound imaging is a technology currently under development that is formed by joining many 2D images recorded when rotating, tilting, or linearly translating the probe. Any transducer used to create 2D B-mode images can be used to acquire slices of 2D images in three dimensions. The mechanical movement can include tilting, rotation, or linear displacement. Usually a motorized transducer is used to accurately determine the relative position of the 2D slice being imaged. Probes for real-time 3D imaging are under development and up to now offline 3D-ultrasound imaging has been developed for clinical use only in the fields of cardiology and gastroenterology.[8]

7.2.2 Magnetic Resonance Imaging

The magnetic resonance imaging (MRI) scan is a radiology technique that uses magnetism, radio waves, and a computer to produce images of body structures. The MRI scanner is a tube surrounded by a giant circular magnet. The patient is placed on a moveable bed that is inserted into the magnet. The magnet creates a strong magnetic field that aligns the protons of hydrogen atoms, which are then exposed to a beam of radio waves. This spins the various protons of the body, and they produce a faint signal that is detected by the receiver portion of the MRI scanner. The receiver information is processed by a computer, and an image is produced. The image and resolution produced by MRI is quite detailed and can detect tiny changes of structures within the body.

There have been a number of specialized advances in MRI technology, one of which is functional magnetic resonance imaging (FMRI) developed in 1990.[8] This is a technique for measuring brain activity. It works by detecting the changes in blood oxygenation and flow that occur in response to neural activity. When a brain area is more active it consumes more oxygen and, to meet this increased demand, blood flow increases to the active area. FMRI can be used to produce activation maps showing which parts of the brain are involved in a particular mental process.

In creating the name magnetic resonance imaging (MRI) physicians wished to avoid using its true name of nuclear magnetic resonance which could cause trepidation. This term was originally applied because when any tissue is subjected to a magnetic field with a defined intensity, the nuclei of certain atoms, themselves being able to be considered as mini-magnets, align themselves to this field. However, because there is no actual radioactivity present in the MRI concept, reference was only made to magnetism itself and the magnetic field measurement. By subjecting these atoms to very low frequency waves, their direction of rotation (or spin) would also change and cause the atoms to resonate at the same frequency as the wave.[1] When the external radiofrequency is switched off, the atoms return to their original state and it is this restitution of the energy they got in the form of a signal which can be captured and measured. Finding the origin of the signal, atom by atom located in space, is the general way an MR image is taken. In organic tissue, hydrogen is the most common atom that has the property of resonance and is the one which is most predominant in human tissue because it is the main element in both water and fatty tissues. Since the percentage of this element differs throughout the body, 3D displays of the body density of water, fats, and other organic matter containing hydrogen can be obtained with MRI.

Although iron is another common element, its existence in particles or pieces of metal (such as those in certain implants and prostheses) and even powders and iron oxides (found in cosmetics) can lead to major distortion of the final image, impeding its interpretation. Since surgical interventions frequently necessitate 3D imaging to allow complete visualization of tumors and other lesions, segmentation of the tissue types in the image must first be undertaken. Manual segmentation gives the best and most reliable results when identifying structures for a particular clinical task. Usually, a medical practitioner with knowledge of anatomy utilizes software to outline or fill regions of target structures on each image slice in an image stack, i.e. a volume. The medical technician will need to mentally reconstruct a structure in 3D because only 2D-image slices can be viewed. Segmentation of each slice requires that each adjacent image is viewed in the stack in order to correctly reconstruct an object in 3D. The task is very tedious and time consuming for an individual, and thus does not serve the need of daily clinical use well. On the other hand, no fully automatic method exists that is able to provide comparable segmentation quality to manual segmentation. Although maximum intensity projections can be used, these are however, inferior to segmentation. A viable alternative may be to apply pulse sequences which would greatly facilitate the segmentation task. There is also a challenge in the case of a patient for whom a determination must be made for the presence of multiple sclerosis because an entire reliable classification of all multiple sclerosis plaques in a 3D image of the brain is required to assess the complete involvement of the brain. This problem has not been fully solved yet. Moreover, it is essential to follow up the change in localization and extent of plaques over many years. This means that it must be accurate and easy to use image registration algorithms for 2D and 3D images.[8]

Tissue classification or other segmentation techniques are not the only ways of separating tissue types in MR images. The Dixon technique, for example, produces separate images of water and fat in tissues which can be important when attempting to solve diagnostic problems such as the retrobulbar spaces. Although these techniques might be based on phase unwrapping of a computed principal phase image,[9,10] they could also be done without phase unwrapping since many of these techniques are computationally demanding and can suffer in the presence of noise.[11]

In some cases, specific contrast agents are used to visualize specific tissues. Hyperpolarized gases can image only the bronchial tree,[12] while aluminum could selectively image the gastric mucosa.[13] Most contrast agents developed in this field are based on the properties of gadolinium. This metallic substance has interesting magnetic properties that could help imaging a specific organ when grafted onto certain substances.[1] Other contrast substances are those that contain an iron core that allows selective imaging of all blood vessels. However, the presence of both arteries and veins in the 3D image usually makes it difficult to fulfill a reliable diagnosis because there are simply too many vessels present. A possible solution is to segment the arteries and veins.[8]

If MRI was more available and more economically viable, it would easily replace most other imaging techniques. At present, however, it is only used for examinations in which diagnosis is difficult (soft tissue such as muscles, tendons, brain, tumors) or in indications for which this method is much more effective or unique (neurology, ophthalmology, cardiovascular, endocrinology, oncology, etc.). It should be noted that MRI neither magnetizes a patient nor does it subject them to any more radiation than from an ultrasound examination and, furthermore, this procedure is also totally noninvasive.[1] 3D localization in MRI is generally achieved by selecting slices in one direction z and then localizing the signal in each slice by means of frequency encoding x and phase encoding y.

7.2.3 CT Scan

Computed tomography (CT), is basically a 3D X-ray imaging system. Since 1895, when Wilhelm Röntgen announced the discovery of X-rays based on his observations of fluorescence and its usage on diagnoses of identified fractures, X-ray imaging has become a very well-known and commonplace modality.

X-rays are high-energy photons that experience insignificant scatter when passing through various media. Usually, X-rays images are shown through a combination of a phosphor screen and a light-sensitive film. However, although this technique provides a good-quality analog image and has been used in mammography and radiography for many years, it is not compatible with the digital storage and transmission requirements of the modern era. Another disadvantage of this standard film-based technology is that it does not provide quantitative data and requires specialized training for accurate image assessment.[2]

Fluoroscopy uses a very similar technique with a slight variation. Fluoroscopy is the method that provides real-time X-ray imaging that is especially useful for guiding a variety of diagnostic and interventional procedures. The ability of fluoroscopy to display motion is provided by a continuous series of images produced at a maximum rate of 25 to 30 complete images per second. This is similar to the way conventional television or video transmits images. While the X-ray exposure needed to produce one fluoroscopic image is low (compared to radiography), high exposures to patients can result from the large series of images that are encountered in fluoroscopic procedures. Therefore, the total fluoroscopic time is one of the major factors that determine the exposure to the patient from fluoroscopy. In fluoroscopy, an image intensifier is used as a transition stage to supply signals to complementary metal oxide semiconductor (CMOS) cameras in order to produce an analog image directly on a TV screen. Since an image in this method is a result of multiple conversions steps (from X-rays to electrons to light to camera display), fluoroscopy gives a poor image quality.

A more advanced alternative to the conventional detection technique uses a digital detector that converts X-ray photons directly into a digital signal. These digital images can be easily transmitted and occupy much less storage space.

Digital X-ray detectors could be used in two different modes: photon counting and integration.[2] In the photon-counting mode, each individual photon is detected and counted when its energy, which is also registered, is higher than the set threshold. In the integration mode, as its name implies, the charge generated by the incoming photon is integrated within a selected time interval. The photon-counting mode is limited to typically about 10^6 counts per second (c/s) whereas it is virtually unlimited in the integration mode.[2] However, in the photon-counting mode it is possible to detect signals down to an individual photon and, as a result, it offers a higher dynamic range. Other advantages of the photon-counting mode include higher detector quantum efficiency (DQE), lower electronic noise, no need for signal digitization, and possibility of energy discrimination.[2] On the other hand, the integration mode can operate at higher count rates and is also more simple and inexpensive to implement.

Standard X-ray imaging suffers from fundamental limitations that makes it only useful for clinical diagnoses in cases of initial screening or simple bone fractures. The main reason for this is the fact that 3D objects are shown two dimensionally. Also, X-ray imaging offers only low soft-tissue contrast and is not very quantitative.

CT, which is actually a 3D extension of 2D X-ray technology, was invented in 1972 and is in widespread use today. The Greek roots of the term "tomography" are "tomo" refers to the act of cutting and "graphos" refers to image. The CT concept was invented by Godfrey Hounsfield in 1972 with the name of computed axial transverse scanning or CAT scan. The scanner was quite similar to other pieces of X-ray imaging equipment with additional requirements for movements and signal processing.

The basic principle behind CT is to project many X-ray beams through the object. The X-ray source is moved around the object in a circular manner and, at fixed angles within the circle, an X-ray beam is emitted and is recorded by an array of X-ray detectors at the opposite side. When the X-ray recording of all projections is completed, based on the X-ray tomographical information, a 3D-tomography image is reconstructed from these projections. CT was the first noninvasive radiological method with which tomographic images of all parts of the body could be generated without superposition of neighboring structures.

Since CT scanners were introduced, subsequent developments in CT technology consisted of attempts to provide faster acquisition times, better spatial resolution, and shorter computer reconstruction times.[2] The main disadvantage of standard CT is that its planar resolution is less than 1 mm, while the axial resolution (or slice thickness) is several mm.[8] Also, each scan lasts about 2 second, and the scans have to be separated by about 6 seconds delays to reorient the X-ray source detector assembly within the gantry to prevent entanglement of cables.[8] This delay is, for some people, too long to hold their breath yet any movement could compromise the quality of the image to the extent that lesions may become obscured.

In 1989, spiral CT was introduced to remove these two disadvantages and it gets its name from the shape of the path that the X-ray beam follows during scanning. The examination table, with the patient on it, moves at a constant speed through the gantry while the X-ray tube rotates continuously around the patient. As a result, the X-ray beam traces a spiral path through the body and allows rapid volumetric data acquisition over a large part of the body. Since a volumetric data set can be acquired during a single breath, it increases acquisition speed and leads to a better imaging of organs that follow respiratory motion. Because an X-ray tube is used continuously for more than 30 seconds in this system, the electrical effect applied to the tube has to be reduced compared to a standard CT. Because of their limited absorption of the X-ray radiation, however, this reduction leads to an increase in the quantum noise of the images which, consequently, must be filtered.[8]

7.2.4 Nuclear Imaging

Nuclear imaging is a method of producing images by detecting radiation from different parts of the body after a radioactive tracer material that is administered. The images are recorded on computer and on film from which the physician interprets the images to make a diagnosis. By detecting these rays, and monitoring their distribution in patient's body, information becomes available for the physician that is not accessible by other methods and can be used in fields as diverse as oncology, hematology, cardiology, and rheumatology.

To inject a radionuclide into the body, a ground (vector) must be used so that the radioactive substance could be labeled to it. These vectors are either salts and radioactive complexes or traditional pharmaceutical molecules (drugs) or biochemical molecules (hormones or antibodies). These radiopharmaceutical molecules are called tracers or radiotracers. The important point in designing such molecules is that it must be ensured that the radioisotope does not break free from its vector through a natural biological process (rapid metabolism), or that it is not eliminated too quickly from the organism.[1]

Next, these molecules enter the body by injection, ingestion, or inhalation and start to emit some radioactive signals, mostly γ-rays (it should be noted that these rays are emitted in every direction). Finally, these emitted signals are recorded on a photographic plate or by specific detectors (cameras). The rays are then selected by a collimator as they pass through, and only those with a direction perpendicular to the detector are taken into consideration. A gamma camera detector composed of a crystal that is sensitive to radiation (for example, sodium iodide), is coupled to a photomultiplier which is responsible for transforming the impact of the radiation into an electronic impulse. A technique called scintigraphy is now employed, which is a form of diagnostic test, whereby the emitted radiation (γ-rays) are captured by external detectors (gamma cameras) to form 2D images similar to an X-ray plate. The difference between this type of imaging and X-ray imaging is that in the gamma imaging method, the source of radiation comes from the substance injected into the patient within whom it has become concentrated in certain tissues. In X-ray imaging, an external radiation source is required during the period of image acquisition and in which the quality is dependent upon the detection crystal's sensitivity and the collimator's resolution. To take a scintigraphy image of the whole body, the detection head is moved along the body to produce a static planar image in a matter of minutes.[1]

Almost all organs can be investigated by employing the nuclear imaging method, and all their functions can be checked without the need for a surgical operation or biopsy. One of the most frequently used investigations is probably bone scintigraphy. When a patient is suffering from bone pain, a whole body image of the patient provides information on bone function that could detect any increase in bone metabolism corresponding to a lesion.

The heart is another organ whose function could be monitored with this technology. This technique, called myocardial perfusion scintigraphy, is based on only monitoring the biological mechanisms of the heart and does not dwell on its shape. Other organs that benefit from the properties of specific radio-labeled vectors are the kidneys. Patients suffering from hypertension and diabetes, as well as those suffering from kidney stones, are subject to routine tests, including nuclear imaging, to provide the urologist with important information concerning blood exchanges and the organ's functionality. The scintigraphic imaging of the thyroid is probably the most widely known specific method to screen for abnormal functioning of the thyroid gland (hyper or hypothyroid), as well as malignant tumors of this gland.

Nuclear imaging cannot be used to obtain images of a damaged organ, since the functional basis of this technique is that the radioactive molecules participate in the cells' biological mechanisms. That is why it could, for example, be used to distinguish between a dead and a live organ which is something that is not possible with other imaging techniques.[1] However, MRI, X-rays, and ultrasound will still provide an image presenting the state or form of a body or an organ, no matter if the individual is alive or dead.

Because the quantities administered in the gamma imaging method are extremely low, less than a billionth of a gram, gamma cameras are able to detect minute quantities of the tracer. X-rays, on the other hand, need a local concentration in order of a tenth of a milligram, and MRI as much as a tenth of a gram, to produce a contrast.[1]

One of the disadvantages with nuclear imaging, however, is that its high degree of sensitivity is inversely proportional to its spatial resolution which makes it difficult to obtain clear images and visible details. This means that the shape and size of small lesions cannot be observed precisely and, to date, it is not possible to distinguish between two neighboring lesions of less than a centimeter in size.[1]

To transcend this limitation, a mixed positron emission tomography (PET)/CT technique is being used, which can specify the location of the source, even if the image of the source remains less than clear. PET is a technique that uses the particular properties of beta-plus $\beta+$ emitters which are injected into the patient in the form of labeled products, binding specifically to the cells for which an image is required. The difference between PET and an ordinary gamma imaging approach is that in PET, positron emitters have the particular characteristics of producing two gamma photons by annihilation, while in single photon emission computed tomography (SPECT) one single gamma signal is emitted. These gamma photons are, however, diametrically opposite to each other so, as a result, this technique needs a suitable imaging tool that complements its power and specific characteristics.

While the SPECT method is ideal for analyzing areas that are well defined and limited in size, such as the heart or brain, the PET camera benefits from the advantage of simultaneous emission in two opposite directions which, in conjunction with mathematical analysis, deduce their origin precisely.[1]

References

1. R. Zimmermann. *Nuclear Medicine Radioactivity for Diagnosis and Therapy*, EDP Sciences, 2006.
2. K. Iniewski (Ed.). *Medical Imaging Principles, Detectors, and Electronics*, John Wiley & Sons, Inc., 2009.
3. K. E. Thomenius. *Instrumentation Design for Ultrasonic Imaging, in Design of Medical Devices and Diagnostic Instumentation*, McGraw-Hill, USA, 2003, pp. 25.1–25.18.
4. E. Krestel. *Imaging Systems for Medical Diagnostics*, Siemens AG, 1990.
5. T. R. Gururaja and R. K. Panda. "Current Status and Future Trends in Ultrasonic Transducers for Medical Imaging Applications," *IEEE International Symposium on Applications of Ferroelectrics*, 1998, pp. 223–228.
6. J. A. Brown, C. E. M. Demore, and G. R. Lockwood. "Design and Fabrication of Annular Arrays for High-frequency Ultrasound," *IEEE Trans. Ultrasonics, Ferroelectrics and Frequency Control*, vol. 51, no. 8, 2004, pp. 1010–1017.
7. F. W. Kremkau. *Diagnostic Ultrasound: Principles and Instruments*, 6th ed., W. B. Saunders, 2002.
8. T. Taxt, A. Lundervold, J. Strand, and S. Holm. "Advances in Medical Imaging," *Invited Plenary Talk in 14th International Conference on Pattern Recognition (ICPR'98)*, 1998.

9. B. D. Coombs, J. Szumowski, and W. Coshow. "Two-point Dixon Technique for Water-fat Signal Decomposition with B_0 Inhomogeneity Correction," *Magnetic Resonance in Medicine*, vol. 37, 1997, pp. 884–889.
10. T. E. Skinner and G. H. Glover. "An Extended Two-point Dixon Algorithm for Calculating Separate Water, Fat, and B_0 Images," *Magnetic Resonance in Medicine*, vol. 37, 1997, pp. 628–630.
11. Q. S. Xiang and L. An. "Water-fat Imaging with Direct Phase Encoding," *Journal of Magnetic Resonance Imaging*, vol. 7, 1997, pp. 1002–1015.
12. P. Bachert, L. R. Schad, M. Bock, M. V. Knopp, M. Ebert, T. Grossmann, W. Heil, D. Hoffman, R. Surkau, E. W. Otten. "Nuclear Magnetic Resonance Imaging of Airways in Humans with the Use of Hyperpolarized ^{3}He,"*Magnetic Resonance in Medicine*, vol. 36, 1996, pp. 192–196.
13. A. Kaspar, D. Bilecen, K. Scheffler, and J. Seelig. "Aluminum-27 Nuclear Magnetic Resonance Spectroscopy and Imaging of the Human Gastric Lumen," *Magnetic Resonance in Medicine*, vol. 36, 1996, pp. 177–182.

CHAPTER 8

Applications of Mechatronics in Medicine

8.1 Introduction

In this chapter, the most important applications of mechatronics in medicine and biomedical engineering fields are presented. These applications include robotics in medicine, smart instruments and probes, and navigation.

8.2 Robotics in Medicine

The idea of using robotics for medical applications was originally conceived and implemented about two decades ago because advances in robotic technology were, by then, sufficiently advanced so as to make it an acceptable and feasible addendum to the field of medical science. Following its introduction, robotic application in the medical field has been used mainly in three specific fields, namely, surgery, diagnosis, and artificial limbs.[1]

The advantages of robotic surgery are that it is possible to operate in a confined space and, because it is minimally invasive, the outcome is generally better.[1] Today, robots are routinely used in heart, brain, spinal cord, throat, and knee surgeries in many hospitals throughout the United States.[2]

Robotics in medicine is also used in diagnosis for which it is not only much more accurate but, just as in surgery, is equally minimally invasive.[1] A good example of this is the robotic capsular endoscope that can be used for making a noninvasive diagnosis of the gastrointestinal tract.

Finally, robotics is used to help restore physical functions by providing patients with prosthetic legs, arms, and hands.[1] An example of this is bilateral robotic orthosis called Lokomat® (Hocoma AG, Volketswil, Switzerland) shown in Fig. 8.1. This device is used in conjunction with a treadmill and a dynamic body weight support to control the patient's leg movements in the sagittal plane.[3–5] The Lokomat's hip and knee joints are activated by linear back-drivable actuators connected to an exoskeleton structure. Passive foot lifters help ankle dorsiflexion during the swing phase. The patient's legs, which are fixed to the exoskeleton by straps, are moved according to a position control strategy with predefined hip and knee joint trajectories.

The following sections provide examples of robotic applications in the medical domain.

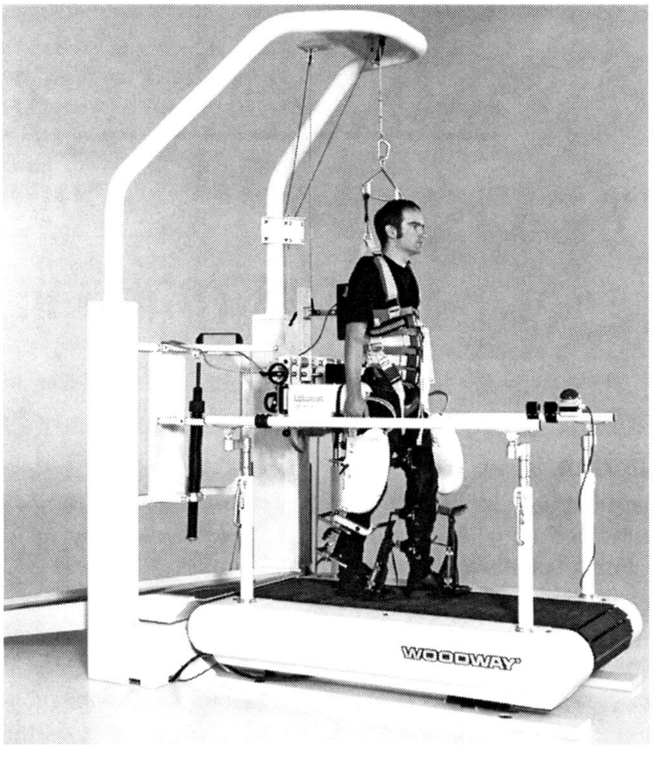

FIGURE 8.1 The Lokomat is a driven gait orthosis with electromechanical drives for hip and knee joint (2 degrees of freedom per leg).[3–5] (With permission of Hocoma AG, Volketswil, Switzerland)

8.2.1 Robots in Surgery

Robotic surgery was first applied in the early 1900s and, with the advent of technology, has developed significantly since then.[6] Procedures are now being performed on the retina, middle ear, brain, and spinal cord, as well as reconstruction of nerves and vessels in the hand.[7] The use of robots in surgery has equipped surgeons with additional tools and has enabled them to fulfill minimally invasive procedures and to perform remote teleoperated surgeries.[8]

In order that these procedures adhere to the strict standards required in all surgical procedures, modern surgical robotic systems are based on the interaction of appropriate hardware and proven software components. Surgical manipulators are the most important hardware components of surgical robotic systems and are responsible for holding, or precisely moving, the surgical instruments under computer control.

The most common kinematic part of surgical manipulators is the remote center of motion (RCM) which is used to orient the surgical instrument and provide its rotational motion about a fixed point in space, usually located on the instrument. Another important hardware component is the image acquisition device, e.g., video, infrared, ultrasound, X-ray, and magnetic resonance imaging (MRI).[9] Of equal importance is computer software since it provides a connection between the data acquired from medical images, sensors and databases, and the physical world of surgical actions.[9] Software is used to plan and execute surgical interventions accurately and predictably, employing both real-time and presurgical information about the patient.[10]

Currently, the Zeus and da Vinci robotic systems are the two most commonly used in current remote robot-assisted surgery. Zeus, developed in early 1990s by Computer Motion, is used in laparoscopic procedures such as general, cardiac, gynecologic, urologic, and pediatric surgeries. Each Zeus system consists of two physically separated parts: the "surgeon side" and the "patient side". The surgeon-side console has a monitor for capturing the surgical process and contains two handles which the surgeons use to control the robotic arms and manipulate surgical instruments. The patient side part has three robotic arms controlled by the surgeon console. These robotic arms can be equipped with a variety of surgical instruments and either 3D video monitoring or imaging microsystems.[11,12]

In 1999, the da Vinci Surgical System was introduced by Intuitive Surgical, Inc. to facilitate delicate and complex minimally invasive operations. The system is comprised of three components: a surgeon console, equipped with a 3D stereo viewer; a patient-side cart designed to hold up to four robotic arms; and a vision cart housing camera control boxes, light sources, and a synchronizer. The system offers the combination of seven total degrees of freedom: insertion, pitch and yaw in the arms and roll, grip, pitch and yaw in the wrists.[13] Figure 8.2 shows the components of a da Vinci Surgical System.

8.2.2 Nano Robotics in Medicine

It is hypothesized that in future the principal focus in medicine will shift from medical science to medical engineering in which the techniques provided from human molecular structural knowledge, gained in the twentieth and early twenty-first centuries, will enable humans to design and manufacture medically active microscopic machines.[14] Within this sphere, nano robotics will mainly be applied in two major areas, namely surgery and constant patient monitoring.[15] However, to fulfill such goals, the feasibility of fabrication and assembly of nano scale parts must first be established. These two capabilities had been demonstrated to a limited degree as early as 1998 through the use

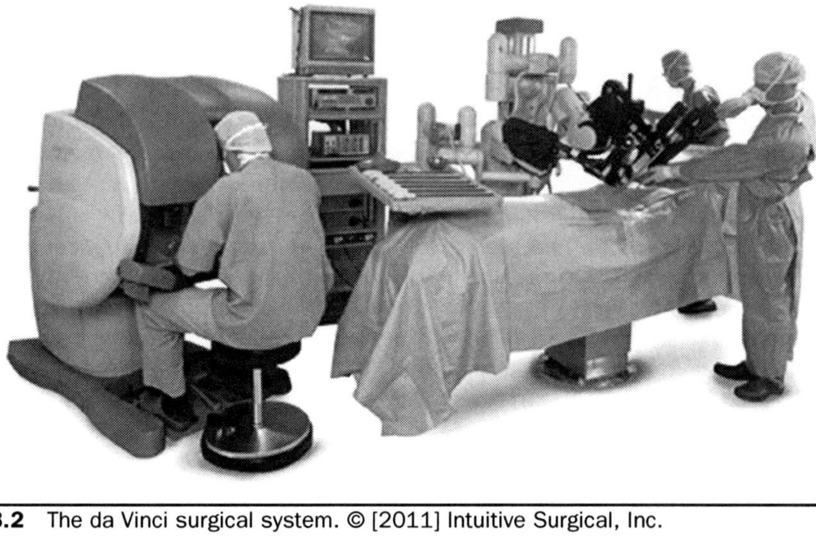

Figure 8.2 The da Vinci surgical system. © [2011] Intuitive Surgical, Inc.

of different approaches such as biotechnology, supramolecular chemistry, and scanning probes.[14]

Developments in the field of bimolecular computing,[16] have proved that processing logic tasks using bio-computers is now feasible and is the first step toward building future nano processors.[17] However, unlike manufacturing larger robots, the greater forces inherent within this environment (turbulent fluid velocities and Brownian motion) are the dominant forces that must be considered.[15] Also, there has been progress in building biosensors,[18] and nano kinetic devices,[19,20] which enables nano robotic operations and locomotion.

8.2.3 Rehabilitation Robotics

One of the most extensive applications of medical robotic technology is rehabilitation that traditionally includes assistive robots, prosthetics, orthotics, and therapeutic robots.[21]

Assistive robots are those which help disabled people to carry out their daily activities and to provide them with a greater degree of autonomy. For example, robot manipulators assist individuals, who have little or no hand function, with essential tasks such as eating and drinking, or prosaic tasks such as opening a filing cabinet. Assistive robotics also includes mobility aides, such as wheelchairs and walkers with intelligent navigation and control systems, in order to help individuals with impaired lower-limb function.

A prosthetic is a mechanical device used for substituting a missing part of the human body and prosthetic related robots are often used to restore lost mobility or manipulation functions. An orthotic is a mechanism that is aimed to assist or support a weak or ineffective joint, muscle, or limb and often comes in the form of an exoskeleton, a powered anthropomorphic suit worn by the patient.[21]

For individuals with disabilities following a stroke, therapeutic robots have the great potential to become valuable tools for delivering neuro-rehabilitation in order to restore limb movement. These robotic therapeutic techniques are used to actively assist and/or resist the motion of the patient. Also, therapeutic robots can be programmed to continuously collect data so that therapists are able to optimize treatment techniques using data acquired throughout the patient's recovery process.[21]

8.2.4 Surgical Training Simulators and Haptic Interface

Training surgical residents adds significant cost to the annual budget of most medical-care institutions. A resident is also more likely to make a mistake than a more experienced surgeon which could result in economic, legal, and societal liability. It has been several decades since flight simulators were used to train airline and military pilots in a virtual reality environment,[21] and it was this precedent that inspired using similar systems in medical applications. Residents are currently trained on different modalities: first on plastic models, next on animals, and finally on human patients. Using a virtual reality environment, however, enables residents, under differing and difficult simulated anatomical case scenarios, to become more proficient and to learn more easily, since any mistakes that are made will not result in any ethical or financial liability.

A typical virtual reality surgical simulator consists of hardware and software. The input data, in some surgical simulators, are gathered only by sensors which show the position of the tools. In more advanced systems, a haptic interface is used

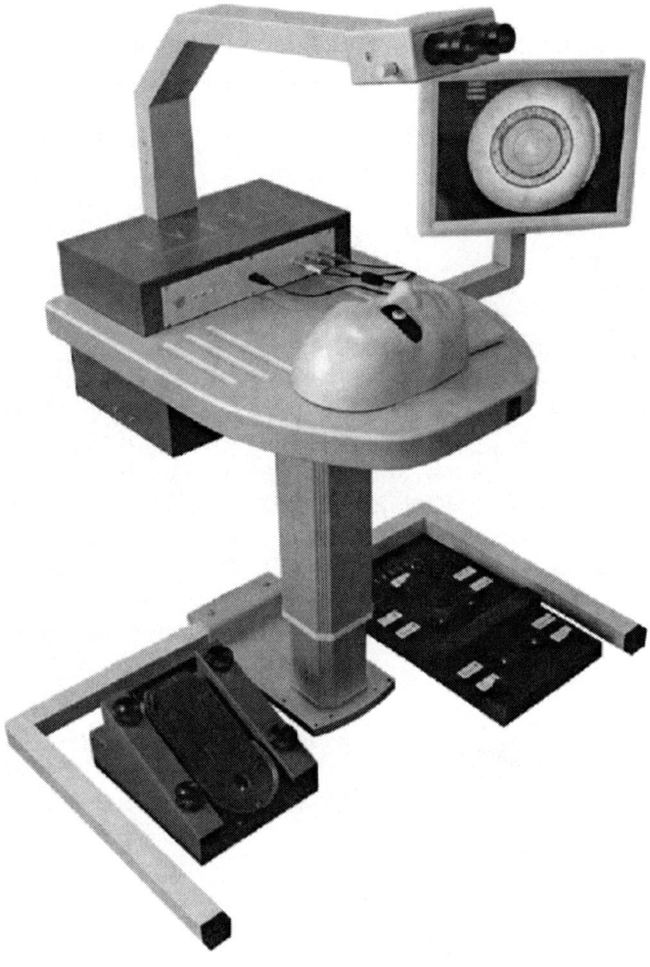

FIGURE 8.3 EYESI, an ophthalmic virtual reality surgical training system, produced by VR Magic. (With permission of VR Magic Holding AG)

which incorporates actuators in addition to position sensors. These actuators are able to generate the appropriate force feedback when the tools interact with the virtual medium.

One commercially available surgical training system, which has been developed for ophthalmic surgery, is shown in Fig. 8.3. In this system, handheld instruments can move freely into a dedicated artificial eye and their interaction with the tissue and ocular structure is simulated and shown simultaneously. During the simulation, all essential microscopic and machine functions can be controlled by means of foot pedals.[9]

Another way to simulate a surgical procedure is to use the surgeon console (master) of any robotic system and a virtual model instead of the patient. In this way, it is possible to connect two or more consoles together so that two or more surgeons can share both the visual view and the haptic sensation of the surgical scene.[21]

At the heart of any simulator is a computational engine, which samples the tool positions as inputs and generates the graphical representation of the surgical scene. It also provides force feedback as outputs, based on a model of the virtual material, and uses both the mass-spring and finite element models to simulate soft tissues. However, the problem is that these models are considered to be an oversimplification of real soft tissue which does, in actuality, exhibit nonlinear, heterogeneous and viscoelastic behavior.[21] *In vivo* measuring of the biomechanical characteristics of soft tissue instead of *in situ* or under postmortem conditions might be a way of solving this problem.[22,23]

8.3 Smart Instruments and Probes

A smart instrument has an embedded or external controller (provided by imaging and/or sensing data) to guide the operation either indirectly (by providing the surgeon with enhanced information on the anatomy or structure of the operating site) or directly (by providing the controller with such information for real-time adaptation to the environment). The block diagram of a typical smart surgical tool used in computer-assisted surgery is shown in Fig. 8.4. As shown in this diagram, unlike the scenario in traditional surgery, a smart system provides a very sophisticated link between one or more surgeons and the patient. In a smart robotic system the traditional surgeon's free-hand techniques, based on hand-eye coordination and passive information from

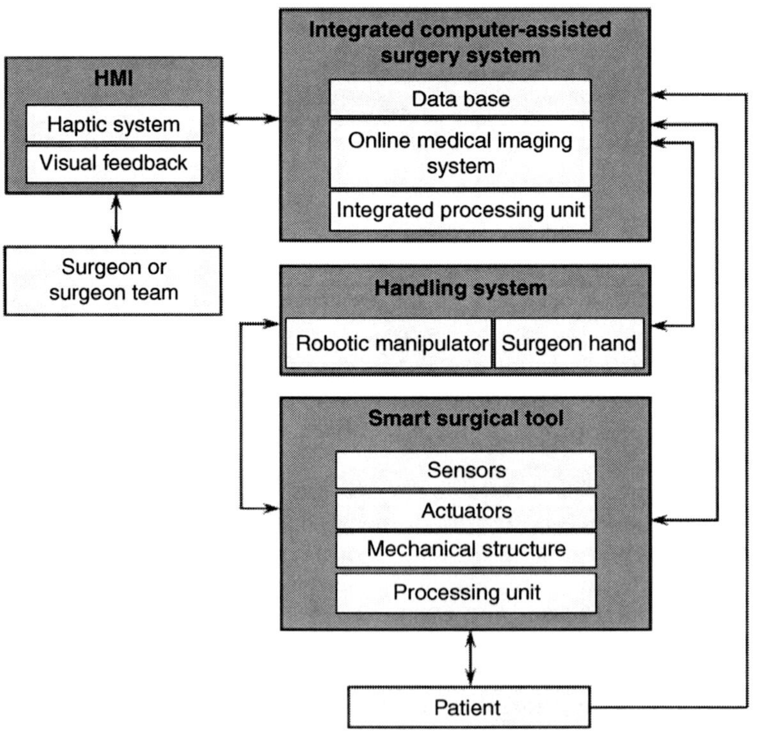

FIGURE 8.4 Block diagram of a smart surgical tool used in computer-assisted surgery.

preoperative images, is replaced by a complex architecture of human–machine interfaces, sensorized and robotic surgical tools, and analysis modules.[6] All these facilities are then integrated so that images taken prior to the operation are matched with those taken during the operation in order to ensure that the surgeon is guided in the best possible way.[24]

There have been many reviews in literature that deal with computer-assisted surgical systems, image guidance architectures, surgical robots for precision procedures, and minimal-access operations of which smart handheld surgical tools is an example.

8.3.1 Smart Handheld Surgical Tools

Smart handheld surgical tools are usually considered enhanced tools which have a certain degree of embedded intelligence and autonomy and are driven by the surgeon's hand. These devices have the ability to support the surgeon by correcting his/her actions, amplifying or weakening his/her interaction within the intervention area, and supplying all-round greater dexterity. A block diagram of this system is shown in Fig. 8.5 followed by a description of two types of handheld tools.

8.3.1.1 Devices to Measure Tissue Properties and Surgical Phenomena

These types of handheld tools are designed to collect data on the mechanical properties of target tissues in surgery. Several graspers have been designed and fabricated that were equipped with different sensors in order to acquire tissue force-deflection properties *in vivo*.[25] The data gathered from such instruments are used to yield more accurate parameters and models for surgical simulators.

Another category of these types of handheld devices is the one designed to measure forces, torques, and related information at the interface between surgeon and tool,[26] or between tool and tissue.[27] These devices are aimed at collecting any data that is representative of the actual surgical performance itself which, in turn, could be used for making an objective evaluation of surgical skill from which design specifications for surgical robots can be derived.[24]

8.3.1.2 Directly Driven Mechanisms

Another class of handheld tools, called guidance systems, is the robotic or passive mechanisms that are directly guided by the human hand. These systems create a three-way mechanical interaction between the patient, surgeon, and ground (via the mechanism) and constrain or modify the surgeon's motion in useful ways.[24] By placing the surgeon's motion in the correct plane using a guidance system, the surgeon can directly control the motion, orientation, and cutting force of the tool. For example, a sophisticated guidance

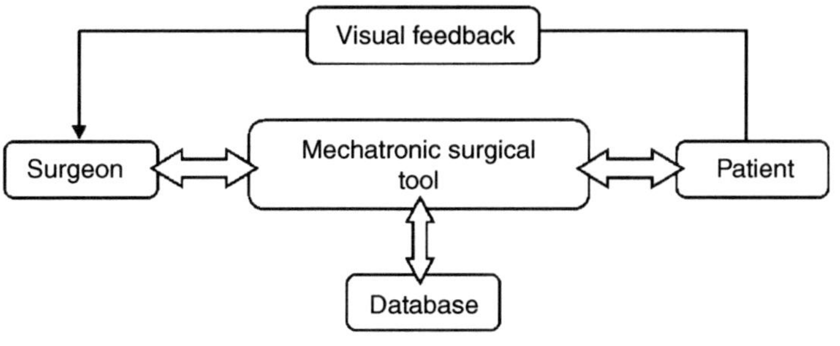

Figure 8.5 Block diagram of handheld surgical tools.

system was developed by Zhu et al.[28] The system had a manipulator to carry the surgical tool and a force-reflecting control handle for the surgeon. The system magnified the force feedback (in addition to constraints and tremor filtering) but, like all such guidance systems, did not allow motion scaling since the surgeon's hand and tool remained connected by a quasi-rigid link.[24]

8.4 Navigation

Navigation systems are used in education and training to provide 3D viewing and virtual planning of instrumentation. These procedures are highly accurate because of the method of registration between the image data, patient tracking, and the tool.[29]

The tracking principle in navigation systems is based on optically measuring the positions of active (luminescent) or passive (IR-reflective) markers that are attached to the tracked object.[29] The attached markers are imaged by either two area-scan or three line-scan camera sensors. With this image data, and knowing the camera parameters, the 3D marker coordinates can be determined. However, there is no redundancy because if the line of sight of one camera is blocked, the tracking process is no longer possible.

The tracking has to be located in a suitable position beneath the area of operation and it is also dependent upon the type of surgical procedure. Optical tracking systems have low update rates and high latency times and, so, are not suitable for demanding tracking tasks such as robot surveillance or tremor control in which fast continuous 3D position data is required.[29]

Tracking can be either active or passive. In active tracking, small RF coils are placed in surgical instruments such as catheters, endoscope, biopsy needles, etc. The position of the coil is frequency encoded by using gradient pulses and the frequency recorded in the coil is analyzed and registered with displayed MR images so, therefore, the location of the coil can be displayed in the image data. In passive tracking methods, some materials are used to determine the displacement of the magnetic spins. Contrast agents can be chemically bound to catheter coatings, for example, in order to intensify large parts of the object.[30]

3D guidance for image-guided therapy depends on the availability of 3D medical imaging modalities. Modern imaging methods such as MRI, CT, and PET generate 3D image sets as part of their standard protocols. Ultrasound has conventionally operated as a 2D modality, but methods have been developed to obtain 3D information from ultrasound.[31]

The most widespread use of 3D image guidance to date is neurosurgery.[32,33] Endoscopic methods with image guidance, to avoid critical structures during the intervention, are also being used in ear, nose, and throat procedures.[34] Cranio-facial surgery procedures using 3D image guidance include osteotomy, bone grafts, and implants. Orthopedic surgery applications include hip, spinal, and knee implants.

Surgical navigation systems, such as magnetic/ultrasound trackers and infrared optical trackers, are useful for tracking the absolute position of objects, instruments, or the patient, within the operating theater. This feature is used for conventional, computer-assisted interventions, where the surgeon performs the action manually while having a better sense of position and orientation of his/her instruments with respect to pertinent structures. This permits a more precise intervention or, indeed, one that was even previously impossible.[29] In a known and restricted application area, one alternative may be imageless navigation. This technique is based on generic anatomical models which are registered with, and adapted to, the patient's individual features by sampling proper sets of surface points. Therefore, the surgical instrument is being tracked intraoperatively and co-displayed with the anatomy.[29] Navigational issues, such as region avoiding or path planning, are decided by the surgeon.

References

1. G. Bekey, R. Ambrose, V. Kumar, D. Lavery, A. Sanderson, B. Wilcox, J. Yuh, Y. Zheng *Robotics: State of the Art and Future Challenges*, Imperial College Press, 2008.
2. International Journal of Emerging Medical Technologies, http://www.medgadget.com/archives/2005/07/da_vinci_robot.html.
3. L. Lunenburger, G. Colombo, R. Riener, and V. Dietz. "Clinical Assessments Performed during Robotic Rehabilitation by the Gait Training Robot Lokomat," *Proceedings of the 2005 IEEE 9th International Conference on Rehabilitation Robotics*, 2005, Chicago, IL, USA.
4. G. Colombo, M. Wirz, and V. Dietz. "Driven Gait Orthosis for Improvement of Locomotor Training in Paraplegic Patients," *Spinal Cord*, vol. 39, 2001, pp. 252–255.
5. G. Colombo, M. Joerg, R. Schreier, and V. Dietz. "Treadmill Training of Paraplegic Patients Using a Robotic Orthosis," *Journal of Rehabilitation Research and Development*, vol. 37, 2000, pp. 693–700.
6. R. H. Taylor, S. Lavallee, G. C. Burdea, and R. Mosges (Eds.). *Computer-Integrated Surgery: Technology and Clinical Applications*, MIT Press, 1996.
7. F. Tendick, S. S. Sastry, R. S. Fearing, and M. Cohn. "Applications of Micromechatronics in Minimally Invasive Surgery," *IEEE/ASME Transactions on Mechatronics*, vol. 3, no. 1, 1998.
8. L. Adhami and E. Coste-Mariene. "Positioning Tele-Operated Surgical Robots for Collision Free Optimal Operation," *IEEE ICRA'02 International Conference on Robotics and Automation*, Washington, DC, USA, vol. 3, 2002, pp. 2962–2967.
9. S. Najarian, M. Fallahnezhad, and E. Afshari. "Advances in Medical Robotic Systems with Specific Applications in Surgery—A Review," *Journal of Medical Engineering and Technology*, vol. 35, no. 1, 2011, pp. 19–33.
10. S. Ramakumar, T. W. Jarrett, and R. Ramakumar (Eds.). *Complications of Urologic Laparoscopic Surgery: Recognition, Management and Prevention*, Norway: Informa Healthcare Location of Publish, 2002, pp. 1–17.
11. J. Marescaux and F. Rubino. "The ZEUS Robotic System: Experimental and Clinical Applications," *Surgical Clinics of North America*, vol. 83, 2003, pp. 1–9.
12. R. A. Faust, A. J. Kant, A. Lorincz, A. Younes, E. Dawe, and M. D. Klein. "Robotic Endoscopic Surgery in a Porcine Model of the Infant Neck," *Journal of Robotic Surgery*, vol. 1, 2007, pp. 75–83.
13. G. H. Ballantyne and F. Moll. "The da Vinci Telerobotic Surgical System: The Virtual Operative Field and Telepresence Surgery," *Surgical Clinics of North America*, vol. 83, 2003, pp. 1293–1304.
14. R. A. Freitas, Jr. "Nanomedicine," vol. 1: Basic Capabilities, *Landes Bioscience*, 1999, http://www.nanomedicine.com.
15. A. Cavalcanti. "Robots in Surgery," *Euro Nano Forum*, Edinburgh, Scotland, UK, 2005.
16. L. M. Adleman. "On Constructing a Molecular Computer," DNA Based Computers, 1995, http://olymp.wu-wien.ac.at/usr/ai/frisch/local.html.
17. M. Hagiya. "From Molecular Computing to Molecular Programming," *Proceedings of 6th DIMACS Workshop on DNA Based Computers*, Leiden, Netherlands, 2000, pp. 198–204.
18. J. Sun, M. Gao, and J. Feldmann. "Electric Field Directed Layer-by-Layer Assembly of Highly Fluorescent CdTe Nanoparticles," *Journal of Nanoscience and Nanotechnology*, vol. 1, no. 2, American Scientific Publishers, 2001, pp. 21–27.
19. R. Stracke, K. J. Böhm, J. Burgold, H. Schacht, and E. Unger. "Physical and Technical Parameters Determining the Functioning of a Kinesin-based Cell-free Motor System," *Nanotechnology*, vol. 11, 2000, pp. 52–56.
20. G. D. Bachand and C. D. Montemagno. "Constructing Organic/Inorganic NEMS Devices Powered by Biomolecular Motors," *Biomedical Microdevices*, vol. 2, 2000, pp. 179–184.
21. J. E. Speich and J. Rosen. "Medical Robotics," *Encyclopedia of Biomaterials and Biomedical Engineering*, DOI: 10.1081/E-EBBE 120024154, 2004, pp. 983–993.

22. J. Rosen, B. Hannaford, M. MacFarlane, and M. Sinanan. "Force Controlled and Teleoperated Endoscopic Grasper for Minimally Invasive Surgery-Experimental Performance Evaluation," *IEEE Transactions on Biomedical Engineering*, vol. 46, no. 10, 1999, pp. 1212–1221.
23. J. Brown. "In-vivo and Postmortem Biomechanics of Abdominal Organs under Compressive Loads: Experimental Approach in a Laparoscopic Surgery Setup," Ph.D. Thesis, University of Washington: Seattle, WA, 2003.
24. P. Dario, B. Hannaford, and A. Menciassi. "Smart Surgical Tools and Augmenting Devices," *IEEE Transactions on Robotics and Automation*, vol. 19, no. 5, 2003, pp. 782–792.
25. A. Bicchi, G. Canepa, D. De Rossi, P. Iacconi, and E. P. Scillingo. "A Sensor-based Minimally Invasive Surgery Tool for Detecting Tissutal Elastic Properties," *Proceeding in IEEE International Conference on Robotics and Automation*, 1996, pp. 884–888.
26. J. Rosen, B. Hannaford, M. P. MacFarlane, and M. N. Sinanan. "Force Controlled and Teleoperated Endoscopic Grasper for Minimally Invasive Surgery-Experimental Performance Evaluation," *IEEE Transactions on Biomedical Engineering*, vol. 46, 1999, pp. 1212–1221.
27. K. S. Morgan, H. M. Hoffman, D. Stredney, and S. J. Weghorst (Eds.). *Medicine Meets Virtual Reality: Global Healthcare Grid*, IOS Press, 1997.
28. W. H. Zhu and S. E. Salcudean. "Teleoperation with Adaptive Motion/Force Control," *Proceeding in IEEE International Conference on Robotics and Automation*, 1999, pp. 231–237.
29. T. M. Buzug and T. C. Lueth (Eds.). *Perspective in Image-Guided Surgery*, World Scientific Publishing Co. Pte. Ltd., 2004.
30. J. G. Webster (Ed.). *Minimally Invasive Medical Technology*, IOP Publishing Ltd., 2001.
31. S. Vaezy and V. Zderic (Eds.). *Image-Guided Therapy Systems*, Artech House, 2009.
32. S. P. DiMaio, N. Archip, N. Hata, I. F. Talos, S. K. Warfield, A. Majumdar, K. Hynynen, et al. "Image-Guided Neurosurgery at Brigham and Women's Hospital: The Integration of Imaging, Navigation and Interventional Devices," *IEEE Engineering in Medicine and Biology*, vol. 25, no. 5, 2006, pp. 67–73.
33. K. Kansy, P. Wisskirchen, U. Behrens, T. Berlage, G. Grunst, M. Jahnke, R. Ratering, H. J. Schwarzmaier, and F. Ulrich, "LOCALITE-A Frameless Neuronavigation System for Interventional Magnetic Resonance Imaging Systems," Proceeding in Medical Image Computing and Computer Assisted Intervention, Cambridge, UK, 1999, pp. 832–841.
34. G. Olson and M. J. Citardi. "Image-Guided Functional Endoscopic Sinus Surgery," *Otolaryngology: Head and Neck Surgery*, vol. 123, no. 3, 2000, pp. 188–194.

CHAPTER 9

Medical Case Studies in Mechatronics

9.1 Introduction

This chapter presents medical case studies in which recently developed devices and techniques were used in various fields of medical practice. These include handheld snake-like robots, smart probes for detecting kidney stones and breast cancer, an ankle-sprain evaluation system, an active prosthetic knee, an instrument for esophagectomy and a smart system for detecting cardiovascular plaque.

9.2 Handheld Snake-Like Robots

Laparoscopy is one of the most common types of minimally invasive surgeries (MIS) because the length of an incision, through which this procedure is performed, is only 0.5 to 1.5 cm. The two most significant drawbacks to this type of surgery, however, are that the surgeon lacks the sense of touch and the instruments used are too rigid and do not have sufficient degree of freedom (DOF). This makes it difficult for the surgeon to perform even common tasks, such as suturing, that require precise and dexterous movements.[1] In an attempt to solve these problems, more advanced robotic units have been designed and fabricated but these, however, are expensive and necessitate lengthy training periods before the surgeon becomes adept in their use. These limitations highlight the importance of fabricating less expensive yet more effective and easier-to-use laparoscopic surgical instruments.

In 2007, Focacci et al. developed and introduced a handheld, lightweight, ergonomic robotic instrument that could be controlled by a surgeon using one hand only.[1] The instrument is equipped with a three-DOF roll-pitch-roll end-effector with a flexibly transferred deriving force. The instrument consists of a handle part and an end-effector. The ergonomic handle part has a control unit that allows direct mapping between the orientation of the handle and end-effector.[1]

Another compact handheld robotic instrument was developed by Mosafer et al. that had all the necessary units attached and, as a result, could easily be moved and replaced during laparoscopic surgery.[2,3] Figure 9.1 shows a final fabricated view of the instrument. The joints are designed in such a way that the end-effector has a bending range of −90 to +90 degrees in both the vertical and horizontal directions.

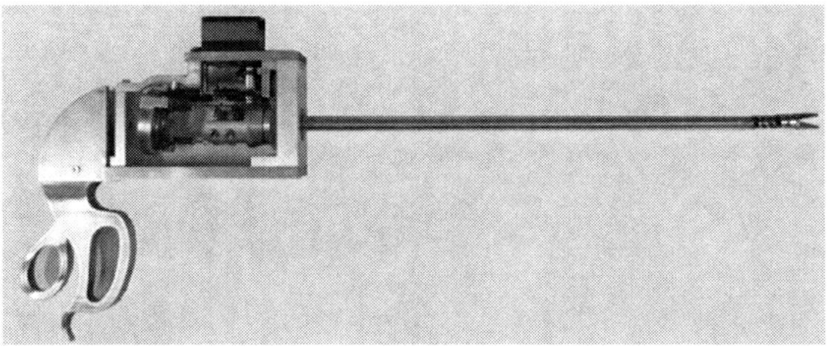

Figure 9.1 The handheld, lightweight, compact robotic instrument. [From Mosafer (2009),[2] used by permission.]

This proposed instrument consists of three main components: wrist mechanism (that provides pitch and yaw rotation between the tool's shaft and end-effector), cable and back-end mechanism, and the end-effector mechanism. To control and manipulate the wrist mechanism and end-effector, a cable actuation mechanism was used. The three different parts of the instrument are described below.

Wrist Mechanism The wrist mechanism, as shown in Fig. 9.2, includes five parallel disks that are joined to each other and provides four DOF. The proximal disk is coupled to the instrument's shaft and the distal disk is coupled to the end-effector support member. The arrangement of the disks is shown in Fig. 9.2 and each is designed to provide a pitch and yaw rotational DOF. The second and the distal disk are able to rotate around a pitch axis, nonparallel to the shaft axis; also, the third and the fourth disk are able to rotate around a second axis, which is nonparallel to either the shaft axis or the pitch axis. Consequently, the wrist mechanism provides four DOF for the surgical instrument.

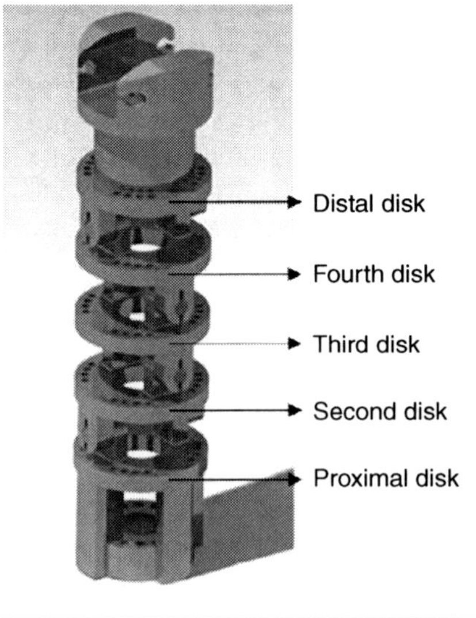

Figure 9.2 Wrist mechanism of the proposed handheld robotic instrument. [From Mosafer (2009),[2] used by permission.]

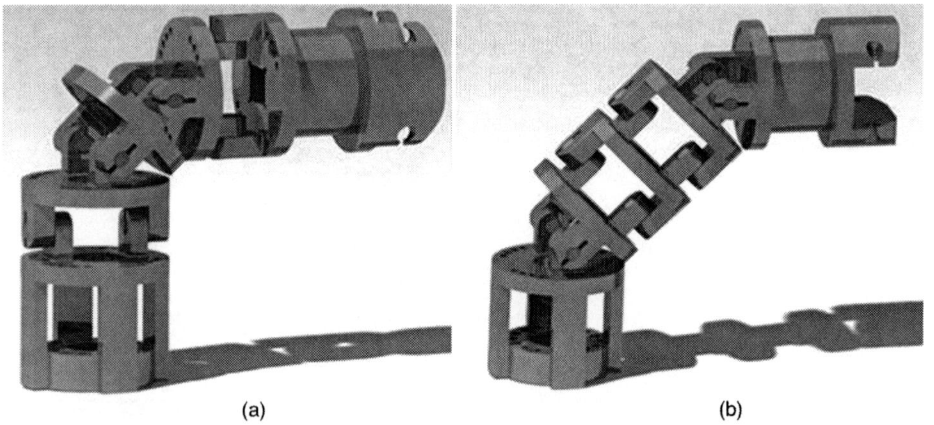

FIGURE 9.3 Combination of two 45-degree rotations of (*a*) yaw and (*b*) pitch. [From Mosafer (2009),[2] used by permission.]

In order to provide a total rotation of 90 degrees in the yaw direction, two consecutive segments of the third disk and the fourth disk were designed to have a rotation of about 45 degrees relative to their adjacent disks as shown in Fig. 9.3*a*. Also, as shown in Fig. 9.3*b*, a combination of two 45-degrees of rotations in the pitch direction between the proximal disk, the fourth disk, and their adjacent disks provide the same results of 90 degrees in the pitch direction. To show the work space of the end-effector of the proposed instrument, Mosafer et al. simulated the instrument's function and considered every combination of angles in the joints. Using MATLAB 7.4, the results of Fig. 9.4 were extracted.

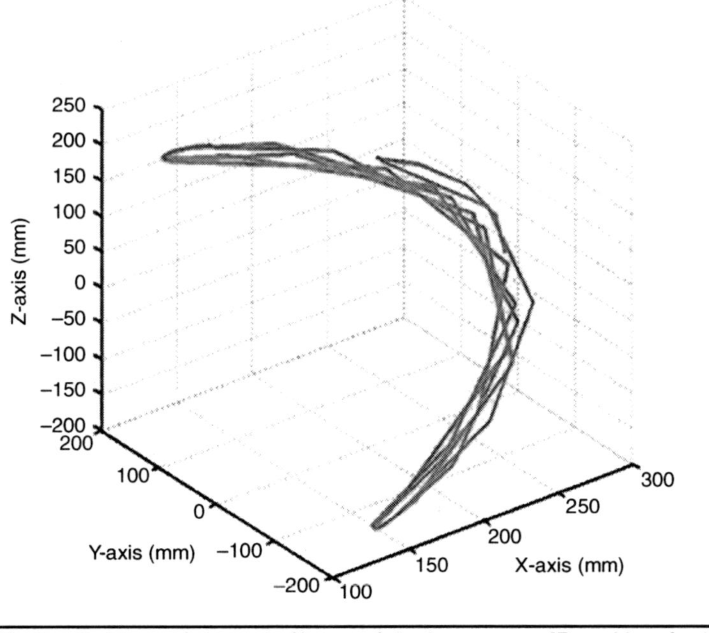

FIGURE 9.4 Different positions of the end-effector of the instrument. [From Mosafer (2009),[2] used by permission.]

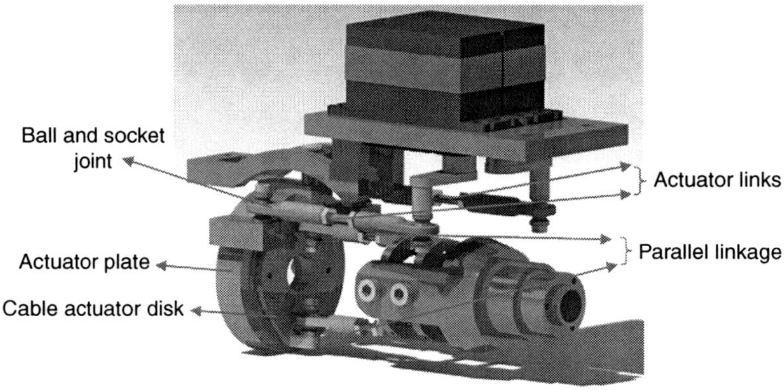

FIGURE 9.5 Designed actuator mechanism to manipulate and control the disks. [From Mosafer (2009),[2] used by permission.]

Cable and Back End Mechanism As previously explained, the wrist segment consists of five disks that are manipulated and controlled via a cable-actuated mechanism. Sixteen cables were used, eight of which are connected to the fifth disk and eight others connected to the third disk. All these cables are connected to a single actuator disk, which is shown in Fig. 9.5.

Manipulating the actuator disk is achieved by means of two ball-and-socket linkage systems. As shown in Fig. 9.6, movement of the links in the same, or opposite, directions would result in the tension of cables responsible for the pitch and yaw rotation. Different combinations of these two types of movements could make any desired orientation of the disk actuator.

End-Effector Mechanism The instrument proposed by Mosafer et al. is equipped with a permanent gripper, as shown in Fig. 9.7. The fifth element of the wrist is considered as the base of the end-effector and consists of two working members, called jaws. A two-part actuator is placed inside the jaws to control the opening and closing of the gripper. Relative movement of these two parts with respect to each other causes the gripper to either open or close. Manipulating these two actuators is achieved via acuation cables

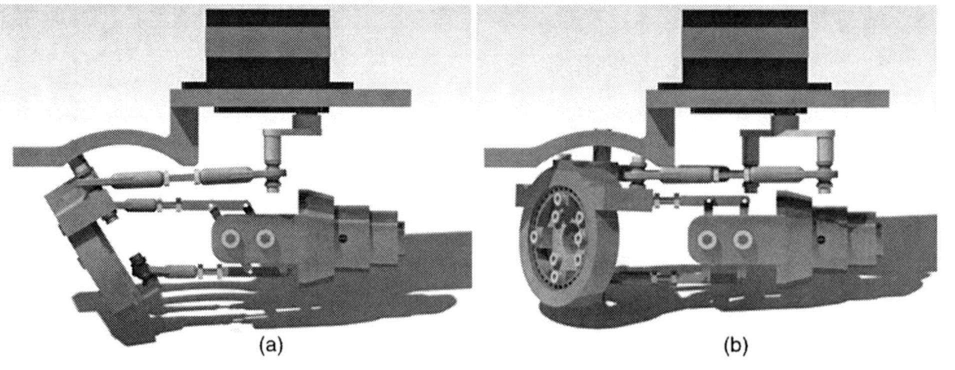

FIGURE 9.6 (*a*) Pitch rotation, and (*b*) Yaw rotation of actuator plate. [From Mosafer (2009),[2] used by permission.]

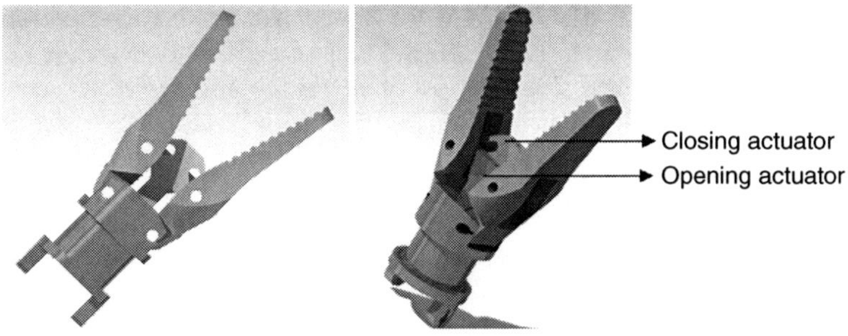

Figure 9.7 The gripper type end-effector of the proposed instrument and its inside two-part actuator. [From Mosafer (2009),[2] used by permission.]

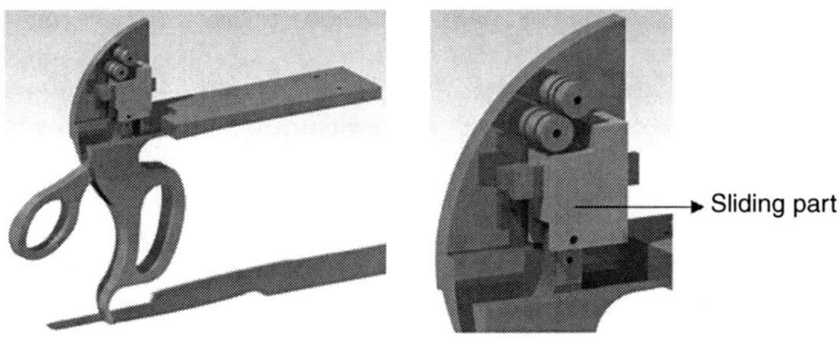

Figure 9.8 The sliding mechanism that changes handle rotational movement to linear displacement of gripper cables. [From Mosafer (2009),[2] used by permission.]

attached to a sliding part that is controlled by the surgeon. The sliding part moves on a rail and transforms the rotational movement of the handle into the linear movement of the opening and closing actuation cables. The handle and mechanism for transfering the rotational to linear movement is shown in Fig. 9.8 and is designed so that a 40-degree rotation of the handle provides a whole range of motion of the actuation cable.

Drive Unit Movement of the handheld robot's end-effector is controlled by two servomotors and a joystick located on the handle. The servomotors are controlled by a microcontroller so that the instrument's wrist orientates in a direction along which the surgeon moves the joystick. A DC motor is then used to rotate the shaft because even if the wrist is orientated correctly, the grasper might be in an incorrect position and unable to grasp the tissue. So, the shaft needs to be rotated in order to place the grasper in an acceptable position while, at the same time, the wrist orientation does not change.

9.3 Smart Probe for Detecting Kidney Stones

A kidney stone is one of the most painful inflictions from which people suffer and is the third most common illness of the urinary system after urinary infection and prostate disorders. Although kidney stones can occur in both men and women, surveys show that they are more common among men.[4] Different approaches are usually prescribed to control and cure the disease. The physician might at first suggest that the patient should go on a special diet, drink a lot of water, and use medication. Failing that, a lithotripsy procedure can be considered. This is a minimally invasive approach in which the urologist tries to find the location of the stone and pulverize it using X-rays and ultrasound. After a short time, the patient usually can leave the hospital and the smashed stone will be excreted through urination. However, the application of this method is limited should the stone be larger than 15 mm and/or consists of material that cannot easily be reduced to smaller particles.[5] In that case, in order to remove the stone, there is usually little alternative other than resort to conventional open surgery. Although the location of the stone is usually predefined by imaging technologies, the surgeon usually palpates the surface of the kidney during the surgery so that, by using his/her own tactile sense, the exact location of the stone is determined. This cannot currently be accomplished using laparoscopic surgical techniques because the surgeon is denied the sense of touch and, hence, would be unable to determine the location of the stone. Notwithstanding the undoubted advantage this technique has over open-surgery, this is still one of the main limitations of this method for which no scientific solution has yet been found.[6] Recently, however, a novel laparoscopic instrument was designed and fabricated by Afshari et al.[6] that can help the surgeon to determine more exactly the location of a stone in the kidney during a laparoscopic procedure.

To simulate whether or not application of artificial tactile sensing could help the surgeon to find the location of the stone, Afshari et al. used a 3D conceptual finite element model and investigated the applicability of the proposed solution. The simplified model consisted of a cube, with dimensions of 7 cm × 7 cm × 5 cm, to simulate the kidney tissue and a stiff object placed inside as the embedded stone. The kidney tissue and kidney stone were assumed to be of elastic and isotropic material with a Poisson ratio of 0.4 and 0.3 respectively, and the elastic modulus of the kidney tissue was assumed to be 2500 Pa.[7] The experimental data that Cohen and Whitfield extracted in 1993 for mechanical properties of different types of stone was used for the elastic modulus of the stiffer object inside the cube.[8] It was supposed that some parameters including kidney surface loading (compression) c, stone diameter d, stone embedment depth t, and stiffness of stone E are the ones that could affect the stress distribution on the surface of the kidney. These were considered as the input parameters and the different values considered are shown in Table 9.1. A schematic of the model, as well as different considered parameters, are shown in Fig. 9.9.

c (mm)	d (cm)	t (cm)	E (GPa)
2	1	2	3
3	1.5	2.5	6
4	2	3	9
5	2.5	3.5	12
6	3	4	15

Evaluation of a New Method for Detection of Kidney Stone during Laparoscopy Using 3D Conceptual Modeling, Afshari et al., *International Journal of Biological and Life Sciences*, vol. 8, no. 1, pp. 56–61, 2012. Reproduced with permission of World Academy of Science, Engineering and Technology.

TABLE 9.1 Values of Input Parameters

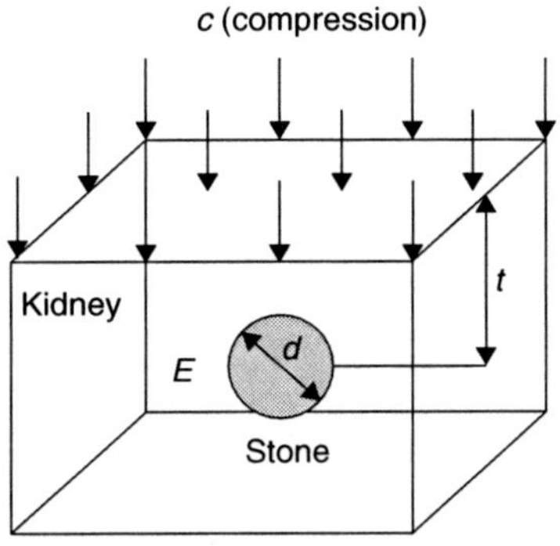

Figure 9.9 Schematic view of the kidney (cube) and stone (sphere) including input parameters. Evaluation of a New Method for Detection of Kidney Stone during Laparoscopy Using 3D Conceptual Modeling, Afshari et al., *International Journal of Biological and Life Sciences*, vol. 8, no. 1, pp. 56–61, 2012. Reproduced with permission of World Academy of Science, Engineering and Technology.

By changing the values of different input parameters, Afshari et al. concluded that the existence of a stone in the kidney changes the stress distribution on the surface of the kidney and it actually increases near the location of the stone.[9, 10] A stress distribution contour graph for one of the analyzed models is shown in Fig. 9.10. In order to detect the exact location of the stone, a path is defined on the surface of the model and the values of stress were extracted. According to this graph, the maximum value of stress will occur at the exact location of the embedded stone.

The graphs displayed in Figs. 9.11, 9.12, and 9.13 show the effect of changing the value of different parameters on the stress contour on the surface of the kidney. Evidently, by increasing the compression of the surface of the kidney, the easier it is to find an embedded stone. Also, the larger the stone, the easier it is to detect. This trend is inversed when the maximum stress value is mapped against the embedded depth of the stone (Fig. 9.13).

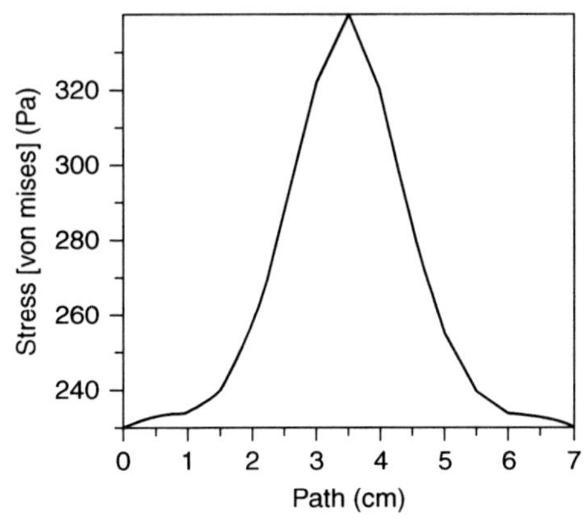

Figure 9.10 Stress distribution contour through the path defined on the surface of the model. Evaluation of a New Method for Detection of Kidney Stone during Laparoscopy Using 3D Conceptual Modeling, Afshari et al., *International Journal of Biological and Life Sciences*, vol. 8, no. 1, pp. 56–61, 2012. Reproduced with permission of World Academy of Science, Engineering and Technology.

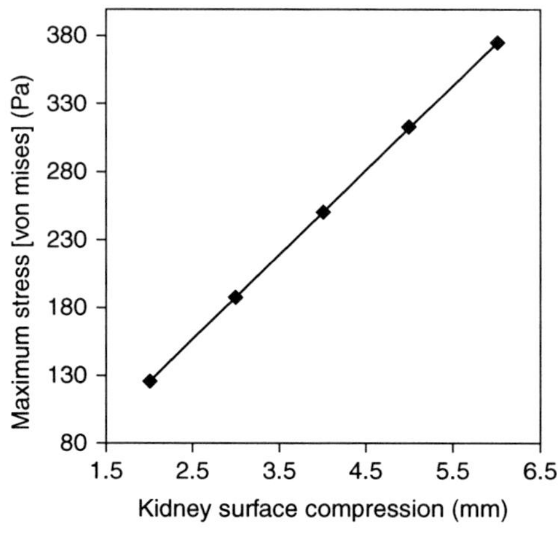

FIGURE 9.11 Variations of maximum stress value due to variation of compression *c*.
Evaluation of a New Method for Detection of Kidney Stone during Laparoscopy Using 3D Conceptual Modeling, Afshari et al., *International Journal of Biological and Life Sciences*, vol. 8, no. 1, pp. 56–61, 2012. Reproduced with permission of World Academy of Science, Engineering and Technology.

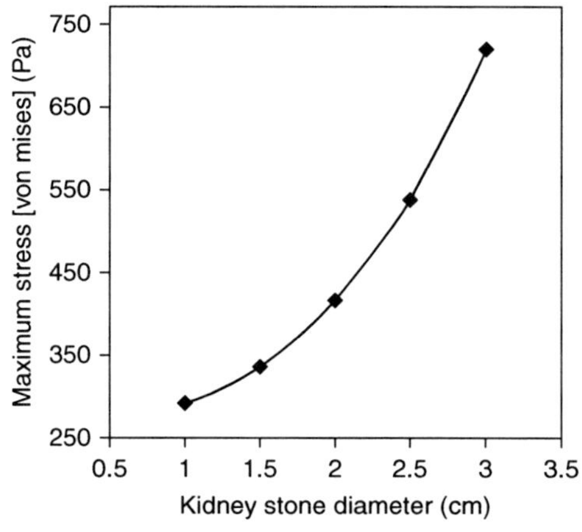

FIGURE 9.12 Variations of maximum stress value due to variation of stone diameter *d*.
Evaluation of a New Method for Detection of Kidney Stone during Laparoscopy Using 3D Conceptual Modeling, Afshari et al., *International Journal of Biological and Life Sciences*, vol. 8, no. 1, pp. 56–61, 2012. Reproduced with permission of World Academy of Science, Engineering and Technology.

Also, it was reported that by increasing the stiffness of the stone, no significant change was observed on the stress distribution diagram of the surface of the kidney.[9]

While modeling and analyzing the results to prove the fact that application of artificial tactile sensing could be a significant advantage during kidney stone removal laparoscopy, Afshari et al. designed an artificial palpation-based system capable of detecting and specifying the location of a stone in a kidney. As shown in Fig. 9.14, such an instrument consists of sensory and mechanical parts, an electrical and data processing unit, and a human interface unit to display the result to the operator.

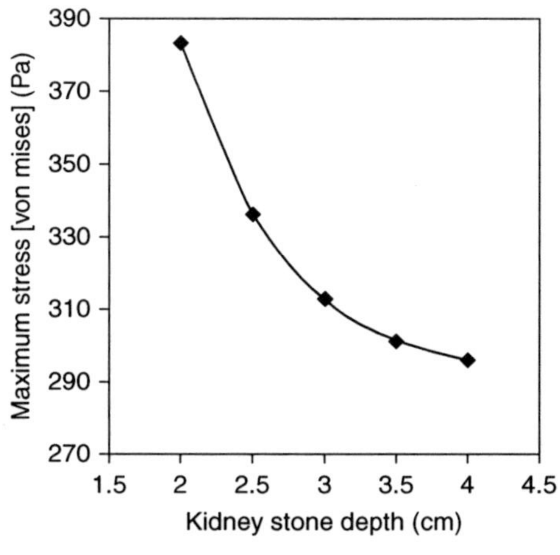

FIGURE 9.13 Variations of maximum stress value due to variation of stone embedding depth *t*.
Evaluation of a New Method for Detection of Kidney Stone during Laparoscopy Using 3D Conceptual Modeling, Afshari et al., *International Journal of Biological and Life Sciences*, vol. 8, no. 1, pp. 56–61, 2012. Reproduced with permission of World Academy of Science, Engineering and Technology.

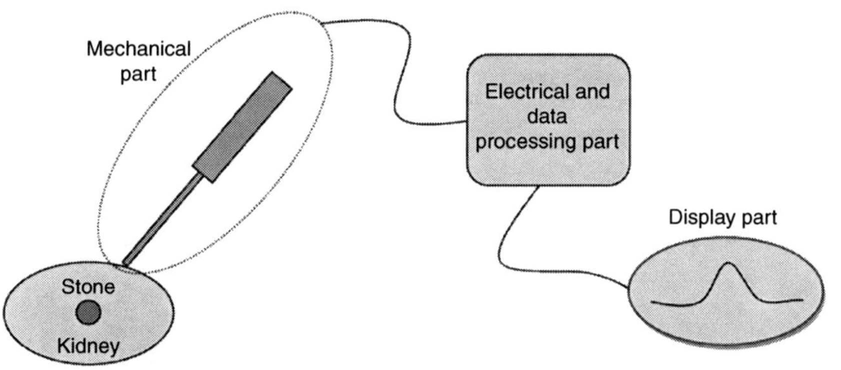

FIGURE 9.14 A schematic view of the novel artificial palpation-based system.
Design and Fabrication of a Novel Tactile Sensory System Applicable in Artificial Palpation, Afshari et al., *Minimally Invasive Therapy and Allied Technologies*, vol. 20, no. 1, pp. 22–29, Copyright © [2011], Informa Healthcare. Reproduced with permission of Informa Healthcare.

The mechanical parts of the fabricated system were mainly divided into the head and the handle. The mechanical parts had to be designed in such a way that they could provide the necessary components of the sensory system in order to easily and accurately receive force and displacement feedbacks. To fulfill the measurement of displacement and force feedback, a Hall effect-based SME1 magnetic sensor and a load cell sensor were used. The flowchart of the designed mechanism is shown in Fig. 9.15 and the final fabricated mechanical parts, as well as sensory parts of the instrument, are shown in Fig. 9.16.

The electrical part, including the appropriate electrical circuits, processes the acquired contact data received from two contact sensors and sent to the display. Two indicators, LD200 and DN10W, receive and transfer the contact data of SME1 and load cell sensors, respectively.

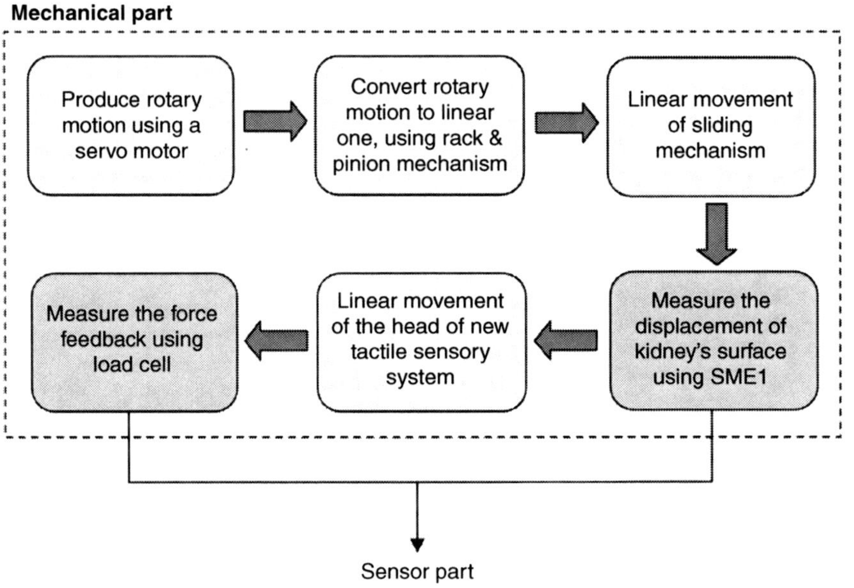

FIGURE 9.15 The flowchart of mechanism used in mechanical part of instrument.

Design and Fabrication of a Novel Tactile Sensory System Applicable in Artificial Palpation, Afshari et al., *Minimally Invasive Therapy and Allied Technologies*, vol. 20, no. 1, pp. 22–29, Copyright © [2011], Informa Healthcare. Reproduced with permission of Informa Healthcare.

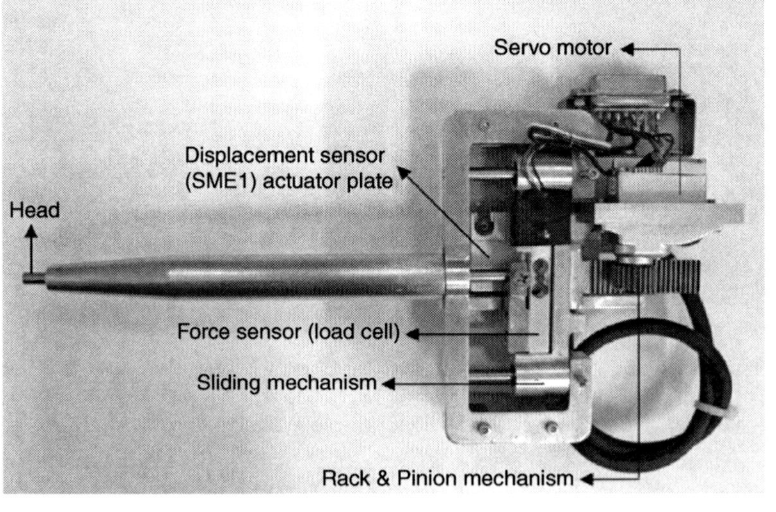

FIGURE 9.16 Different components of mechanical parts of the system as well as two sensors used.

Design and Fabrication of a Novel Tactile Sensory System Applicable in Artificial Palpation, Afshari et al., *Minimally Invasive Therapy and Allied Technologies*, vol. 20, no. 1, pp. 22–29, Copyright © [2011], Informa Healthcare. Reproduced with permission of Informa Healthcare.

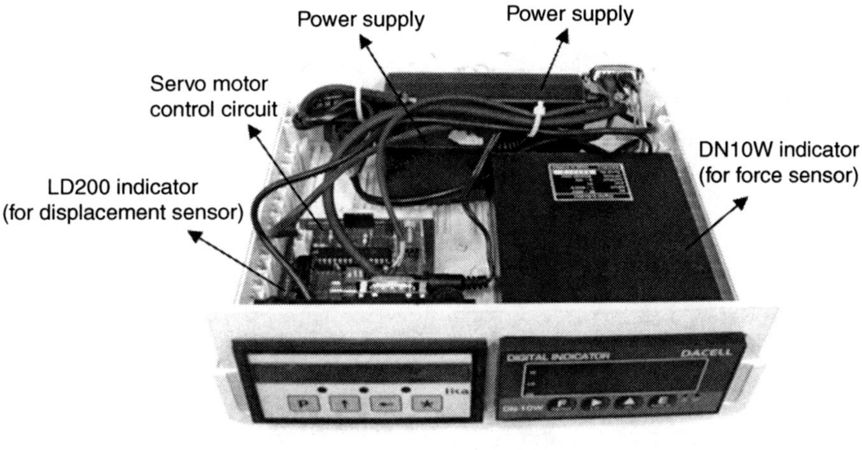

FIGURE 9.17 Different components of the electrical part of the system.
Design and Fabrication of a Novel Tactile Sensory System Applicable in Artificial Palpation, Afshari et al., *Minimally Invasive Therapy and Allied Technologies*, vol. 20, no. 1, pp. 22–29, Copyright © [2011], Informa Healthcare. Reproduced with permission of Informa Healthcare.

Tactile data is transmitted between the mechanical part and the electrical part via the transmission cable. A view of a fabricated electrical part is shown in Fig. 9.17.

Finally, to show the results in a more interpretable way, the display system was designed using Lab View 8.5 software.

To determine whether or not the function of the fabricated system agrees with the model's results, an experimental setup was prepared by Afshari et al.[6] A number of different models were constructed to simulate the existence of a kidney stone using a sheep's kidney which contained a hard object having a diameter of 1.5 cm and depth of 2.5 cm. Then, to simulate the physical examinations that a surgeon executes during open kidney stone removal surgeries, the model surface was scanned by the head of the new tactile sensory system on a line. In fact, the mechanical part of the new tactile sensory system was held by the user and the surfaces of the models made contact with the head of the instrument on a line passing over the simulated stone. Figure 9.18 shows the final fabricated system during the experiment.

Results Figure 9.19 shows the result obtained by performing an experiment on one of the constructed models. The simulated stone was placed in the middle of the experimental model.

The horizontal axis shows the line that the instrument has followed. The vertical axis is the processed outputs of the sensors which are proportional to the force feedback (the force applied by the surface of the constructed model to the active area of the load cell) and the displacement feedback (the displacement exerted to the surface of kidney). In fact, a new stiffness parameter was defined, which is the value of force feedback divided by the displacement feedback.

It should be noted that the point at which the stiffness graph attains its maximum value is the exact location of the stone. To prove the independency of the obtained result to the location of the stone, its place was moved to the left and right of the first experimental model. The stiffness graphs for these two cases are illustrated in Figs. 9.20 and 9.21 from

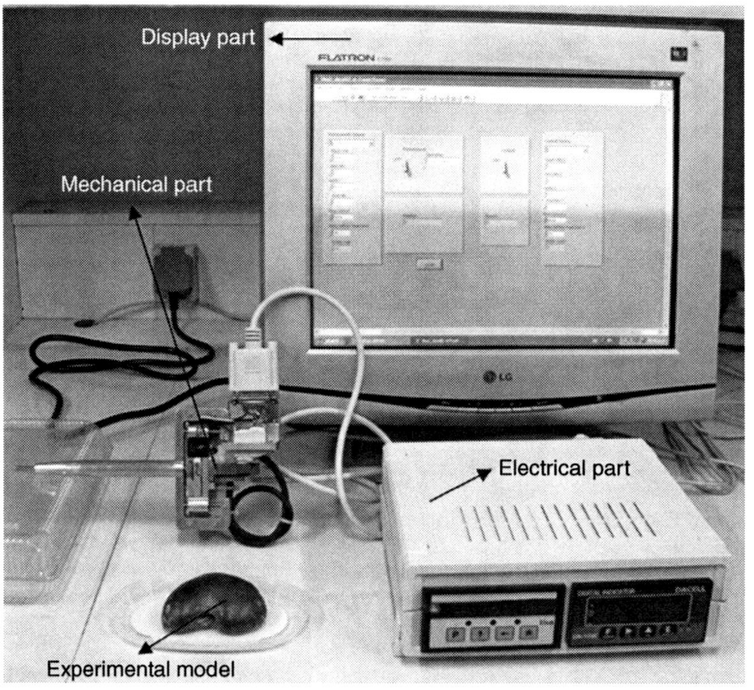

Figure 9.18 The final fabricated system including different parts and the setup of the experiment. Design and Fabrication of a Novel Tactile Sensory System Applicable in Artificial Palpation, Afshari et al., *Minimally Invasive Therapy and Allied Technologies*, vol. 20, no. 1, pp. 22–29, Copyright © [2011], Informa Healthcare. Reproduced with permission of Informa Healthcare.

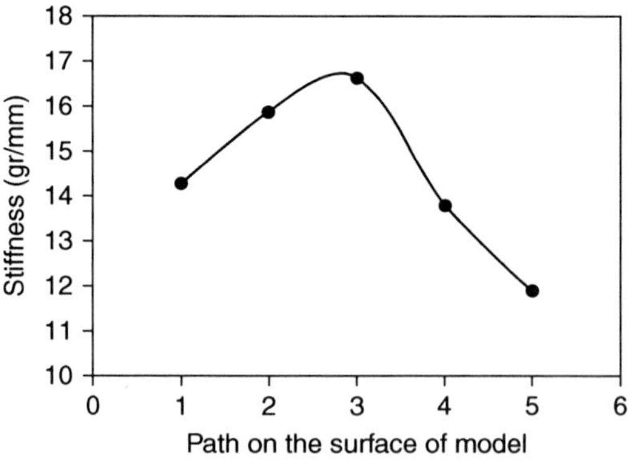

Figure 9.19 Experimental result for a model with a simulated stone at the middle of it. Design and Fabrication of a Novel Tactile Sensory System Applicable in Artificial Palpation, Afshari et al., *Minimally Invasive Therapy and Allied Technologies*, vol. 20, no. 1, pp. 22–29, Copyright © [2011], Informa Healthcare. Reproduced with permission of Informa Healthcare.

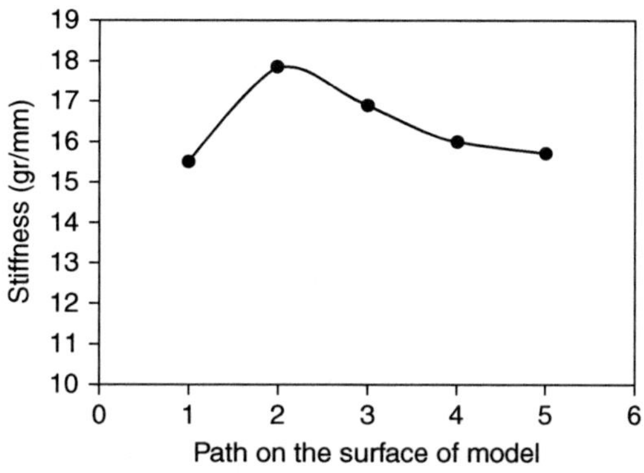

Figure 9.20 Experimental result for a model with the left simulated stone.

Design and Fabrication of a Novel Tactile Sensory System Applicable in Artificial Palpation, Afshari et al., *Minimally Invasive Therapy and Allied Technologies*, vol. 20, no. 1, pp. 22–29, Copyright © [2011], Informa Healthcare. Reproduced with permission of Informa Healthcare.

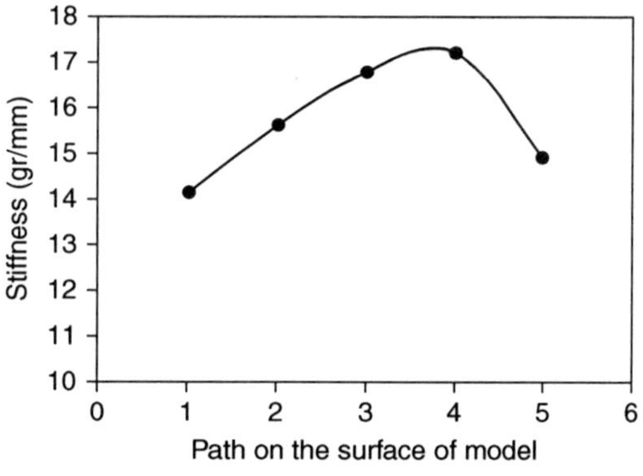

Figure 9.21 Experimental result for a model with the right simulated stone.

Design and Fabrication of a Novel Tactile Sensory System Applicable in Artificial Palpation, Afshari et al., *Minimally Invasive Therapy and Allied Technologies*, vol. 20, no. 1, pp. 22–29, Copyright © [2011], Informa Healthcare. Reproduced with permission of Informa Healthcare.

which it can be seen that the point with the maximum stiffness also moved to the left and right correspondingly.

According to these graphs, Afshari et al. concluded that not only was their new tactile sensory system able to detect the presence of a stone embedded in the experimental models, but it could also be used to determine its exact location.[6]

9.4 Smart Probe for Breast Cancer

The existence of a mass in the breast organ is one of the most common diseases among women. Many lives can be saved each year by being screened for diseases. This is especially true for breast cancer because early detection, while tumors are still small in size and confined to the breast, can save thousands of hours of hospitalization time.[11] One of the most popular breast cancer diagnostic tests is the self-breast examination (SBE) which, for some patients, is preferable to imaging procedures. For example, 12 to 15 percent of cancers that were detected by palpation were not diagnosed through mammography.[12] Clinical breast examination (CBE), ultrasound, mammography, and magnetic resonance imaging (MRI) are the more developed techniques of breast examination used by specialists today.[13] However, the main limitation of these methods are that they require the intervention of well-trained radiologists or surgeons to firstly determine the existence of breast abnormalities and then to provide documentation and detailed analysis. Unlike most conventional techniques, comparing the difference between the stiffness of a mass and its surrounding tissue is a novel idea that is being developed as a new method for testing the breast organ.[14] This is a totally noninvasive technique that avoids potentially harmful exposure to magnetic fields, electromagnetic radiation, and sound waves.[15]

A new method for determining the properties of a mass present in soft tissue is artificial tactile sensing.[16] Recently, Mojra et al. developed a novel tactile sensing robot called "Robotic Tactile Breast Mass Identifier (Robo-Tac-BMI)" that is highly capable of manipulating the end-effecter's movement and which, using a real test tissue model, was used to simulate the palpation of a surgeon during a CBE.[17,18,19]

A Novel Robotic Mass Detector Equipped with Artificial Tactile Sensing

Numerical Method The anatomy of the breast organ consists of three major layers of tissue: skin, fat, and glandular.[20] It was assumed that these three biological tissues and mass would follow the elastic and isotropic behavior. In Fig. 9.22, *a* shows the simplified model including a circular solid tumor in the glandular tissue as an abnormality of the breast, and *b* shows the meshed form of the model developed using ANSYS software (Release 10).

In this model, in addition to the three layers, abnormality of breast tissue is investigated by inserting a circular solid tumor in the glandular tissue. Geometrical parameters of this model are listed in Table 9.2 and mechanical parameters of the reference breast model are listed in Table 9.3.

Since the pectoralis muscle located in the base of the breast tissue restricts the movement of the model in the vertical direction, the base line of the model was assumed to be fixed and used as the reference from which the height parameter of each point is measured.[19] By doing this, it was possible to avoid rigid body motion and solve the problem statically.

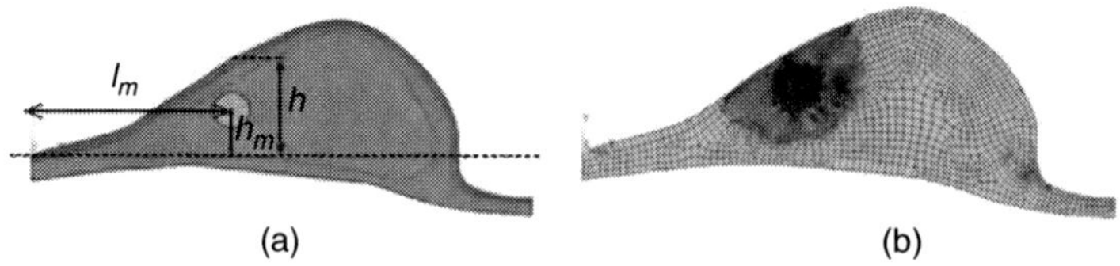

Figure 9.22 (*a*) A simplified model including a circular solid tumor in the glandular tissue as an abnormality of the breast, and (*b*) The meshed form of the model developed using ANSYS software (Release 10).

A Novel Robotic Tactile Mass Detector with Application in Clinical Breast Examination, Mojra et al., *Minimally Invasive Therapy and Allied Technologies*, In Press, Copyright © [2011], Informa Healthcare. Reproduced with permission of Informa Healthcare.

Breast	width (w) (x-dir)	230 mm
	height (y-dir)	70 mm
	fat thickness (t_{int})	5-10 mm
Mass	radius (r)	10 mm
	height from the base line (h_m)	35 mm
	l_m	110 mm
	h	55 mm

A Novel Robotic Tactile Mass Detector with Application in Clinical Breast Examination, Mojra et al., *Minimally Invasive Therapy and Allied Technologies*, In Press, Copyright © [2011], Informa Healthcare. Reproduced with permission of Informa Healthcare.

Table 9.2 Geometrical Parameters of the Reference Breast Model[20,21]

Elastic Modulus	E_{skin}	12 kPa
	E_{fat}	4.8 kPa
	E_{gland}	19.2 kPa
	E_{mass}	57.6 kPa
Poisson's Ratio	$\nu_{skin\text{-}fat\text{-}gland}$	0.49
	ν_{mass}	0.3

A Novel Robotic Tactile Mass Detector with Application in Clinical Breast Examination, Mojra et al., *Minimally Invasive Therapy and Allied Technologies*, In Press, Copyright © [2011], Informa Healthcare. Reproduced with permission of Informa Healthcare.

Table 9.3 Mechanical Parameters of the Reference Breast Model[21, 22]

To perform a thorough analysis of the problem, the effect of the following parameters was investigated:

- Tissue compression in abnormal mass detection.
- Depth of the embedded object's center from the base line h, since there is a probability of the existence of a mass in different depths of the breast. The depth from the base line is shown in Table 9.4.
- Mass diameter d. It should be noted that mass effects on the surface of the tissue in CBE changes markedly with the mass size. Table 9.5 shows different values of the diameter considered for the tumor.

By modeling a number of different cases, including the mechanical and geometrical parameter variations mentioned in Tables 9.2 to 9.5, it was concluded that the stress

h_m(mm)	10	15	25	30	35

From Mojra (2011),[18] used by permission.

Table 9.4 Mass Depth Variations

d (mm)	2	5	10	15	20	25

From Mojra (2011),[18] used by permission.

Table 9.5 Mass Diameter Variations

distribution on the contact surface of the model, called the tactile image, could show the effects of existence of an embedded object. As shown in Fig. 9.23*a*, a nonuniform stress distribution demonstrates signs of an embedded object.[19] Also, in stress graphs taken along a defined path on the surface of the models, there is an increase (overshoot) in the amount of stress that demonstrates the existence of a mass. In Fig. 9.23*b*, D_m is the period of increase in stress graph. As can be seen from Fig. 9.23*b*, the overshoot of the graph, which occurs for almost all mass depths and diameters, not only confirms the existence of a mass but also locates its position. The reason for this is that the position of the summit in each graph coincides with the center of the mass in the tissue.[19]

While a surgeon is palpating to detect a mass, the two major parameters that govern the ease or difficulty of detection are its depth and size.

The stress graphs for different values of mass depth from Table 9.4 are shown in Fig. 9.24 where it can be seen that when the mass depth increases, maximum stress in the abnormal region decreases significantly.

Moreover, in Fig. 9.24, when noting the rate of reduction of maximum stress, it is evident from Fig. 9.25 that the rate is not linear. The reason for this is that D_m increases markedly as the mass moves deeper in the breast and it is known that tissue in the deeper parts of the breast is preponderantly more glandular in nature. Consequently, the mass would tend to blend in with the surrounding tissue making it less easy to localize and is one of the major problems that occur in the palpation of deeply located masses during a CBE procedure.[18]

Because early detection of breast disease is greatly dependent on the detection of masses with smaller diameters, the effect of a wide range of mass diameters ranging from less than 10 mm up to 25 mm was investigated (see Table 9.5). Figure 9.26 displays the stress graphs plotted for different diameters of a mass from which it can be concluded that, for small masses having a diameter of less than 1 cm on the outer surface of the breast, the effect is negligible. This would tend to confirm the lack of ability of a surgeon to detect the early stages of breast diseases.[22] Table 9.6 shows the nonlinearity of stress variations for different dimensions and ratio of the maximum stress for each mass in comparison with a situation in which no mass present. The comparison clearly shows that for mass diameters of less than 10 mm there is no significant difference between maximum stresses.[18]

Experimental Method A tactile sensing robot named "Robotic Tactile Breast Mass Identifier (Robo-Tac-BMI)" was designed and fabricated by Mojra et al.[21] and is shown in Fig. 9.27. It mainly consists of an indentation probe controlled by a robotic system and a visualization interface and, to have easy access to the whole chest area of a patient, the robotic system was designed based on a SCARA (Selective Compliant Articulated Robot Arm) mechanism. The robot contains a vertical shaft for the overall height adjustment of the device, which is driven by a 12-V DC motor. There is also a jointed two-link arm layout that allows the arms to extend into confined areas and then retract or "fold up" out of the way. Two incremental rotary encoders were used to sense and specify the position and orientation of the end-effecter with respect to a defined known reference.

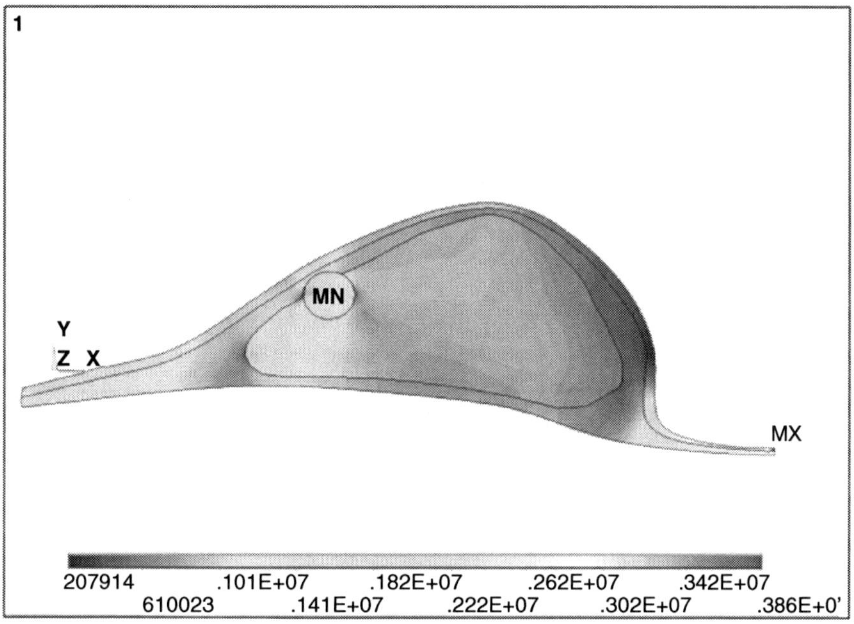

(a)

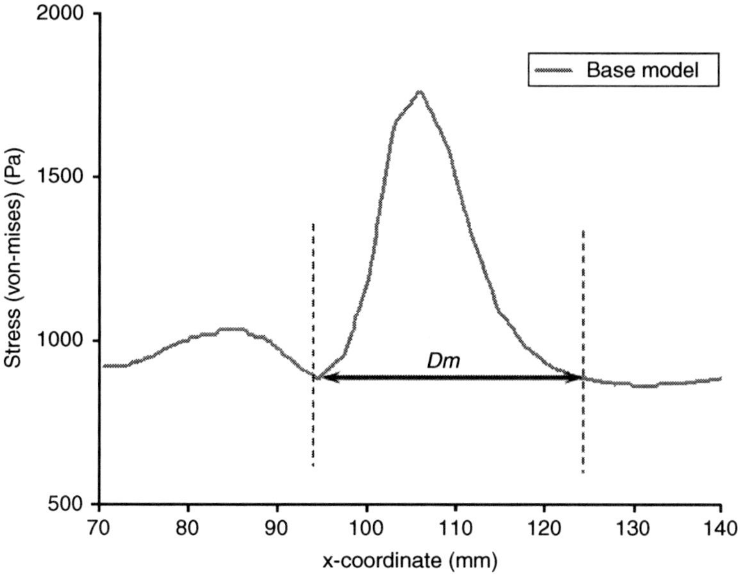

(b)

Figure 9.23 (*a*) Tactile image for the case that the tumor is located 35 mm above the base line, and (*b*) Stress graph of the base model.

A Novel Robotic Tactile Mass Detector with Application in Clinical Breast Examination, Mojra et al., *Minimally Invasive Therapy and Allied Technologies*, In Press, Copyright © [2011], Informa Healthcare. Reproduced with permission of Informa Healthcare.

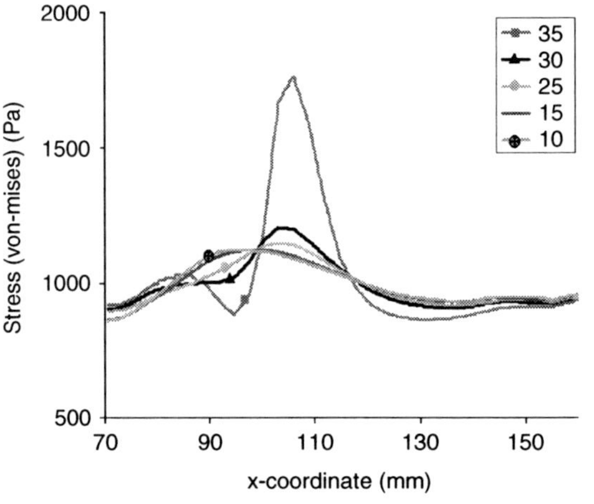

FIGURE 9.24 Stress graphs for different values of mass depth. [From Mojra (2011),[18] used by permission.]

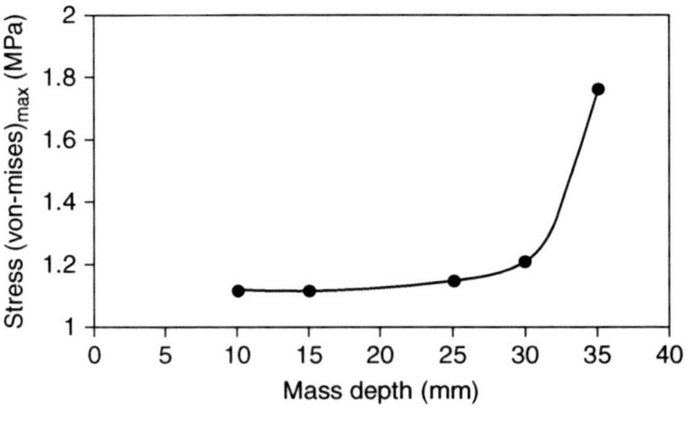

FIGURE 9.25 Maximum stress plotted against mass depth. [From Mojra (2011),[18] used by permission.]

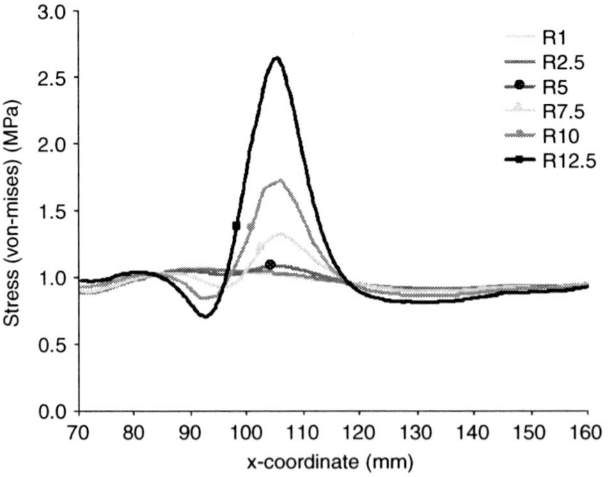

FIGURE 9.26 Stress graphs for different values of the mass radius. [From Mojra (2011),[18] used by permission.]

Mass Diameter (*d*) (mm)	2	5	10	15	20	25
S (von-Mises) $_{max}$ (MPa)	1.07	1.06	1.08	1.32	1.73	2.64
Ratio ($S_{mass}/S_{no\ mass}$)	1.02	1.01	1.04	1.27	1.65	2.53

From Mojra (2011),[18] used by permission.

Table 9.6 Maximum Stress Experienced by Different Size of the Mass Compared to the Healthy Breast

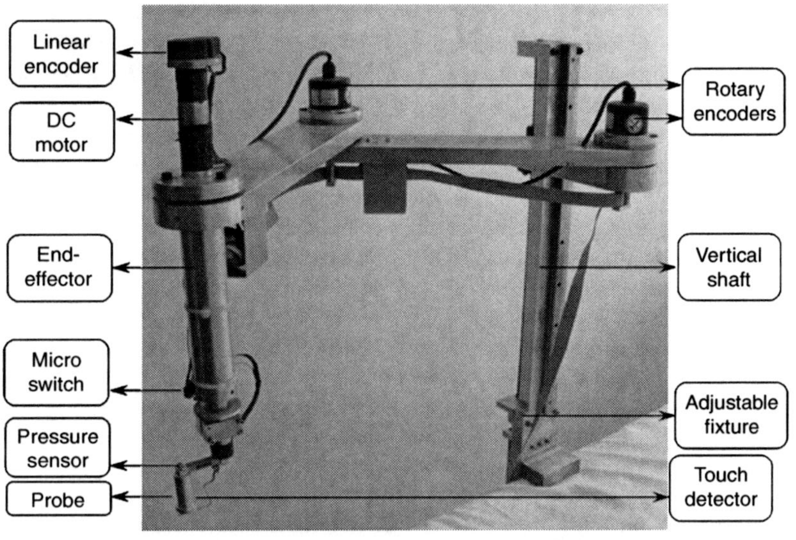

Figure 9.27 Fabrication of a tactile sensing robot called "Robotic Tactile Breast Mass Identifier (Robo-Tac-BMI)".

A Novel Robotic Tactile Mass Detector with Application in Clinical Breast Examination, Mojra et al., *Minimally Invasive Therapy and Allied Technologies*, In Press, Copyright © [2011], Informa Healthcare. Reproduced with permission of Informa Healthcare.

An incremental linear encoder provides a linear output characteristic with displacement which is proportional to the supply voltage. The probe manipulated by the robot consists of a pressure sensor and a touch detector mechanism. As a result of breast tissue complexities, a very precise sensor, "Minigram Beam Load Cell: (MBL)," was used to detect abnormalities underlying several layers.

The probe's testing area has a circular shape and is completely flat and smooth. Three different diameters for the probe: 1 cm, 2 cm, and 3 cm were considered. The whole system is controlled by an electronic board including a PIC microcontroller with serial programming capability (to receive and process the data sent from the sensor), a RAM IC, a 10-bit Counter IC (to decrease pulse numbers of the linear encoder mounted on the end-effecter shaft so that the microcontroller can count encoder pulse numbers), two 8-bit Counter ICs (to address RAM cells), a Voltage Regulator IC (to automatically maintain a constant voltage level), a motor driver IC, USB to RS-232 converter IC (to convert the USB port data of the computer to a RS-232 serial port data), a switch (inserted to provide the possibility of resetting the Robo-Tac-BMI output data and position for each patient), an on/off switch, and a 220V/12V voltage converter adaptor.[17]

The robot is designed to provide the ability for the operator to readily control and manipulate the vertical movement of the whole system and also adjust the height of the Robo-Tac-BMI for patients with different anatomical features. It also provides vertical movement (displacement) of the end-effecter on the tissue surface regarding the touch point, the start, and end point of the end-effecter's displacement course, speed of the end-effecter vertical movement, and step of data acquisition during the course of compression and tension.

In addition, the system gives the operator the opportunity to set the coordinate of the original point of each breast, so that the coordinates of all other testing points would be relative to this point. In fact, the nipples were chosen as the origin of both breasts. Physicians divide each breast into 12 equal sections and express the angular position of a point as the hours of the clock with respect to the nipple.

Breast anatomy is complicated and the soft tissue not only varies considerably between each individual but may also be different, quadrant by quadrant, in each particular individual as well.[23] The problem becomes even more compounded when considering the fact that even for a single breast, the variation in tissue is considerable. As a result, it becomes virtually impossible to find a single criterion that can demonstrate breast abnormalities for all patients. In the research done by Mojra et al., the key point they proposed for making a precise decision was the comparison of the symmetrical points of both breasts. Axis of symmetry was considered to be the sternum of the patient.

The Robo-Tac-BMI was programmed to have an output of the force sensed by the load cell in the loading-unloading process in different steps of displacement (compression-tension). According to these loading/unloading graphs, three types of stiffness were measured for each test point:[21]

1. *Start point stiffness (SPS)*, which is defined as the slope of the loading curve at the start point of the curves and is a valuable parameter when the mass is located near the surface of the tissue.
2. *Average stiffness* (*AvS*), which is defined as the average of the stiffness of steps of data acquisition during the course of compression. This parameter is of more significance when the mass is located deeply and does not have a noticeable effect on the surface.
3. *Normalized stiffness* (*normS*), which is defined as the ratio of the start point stiffness to the average stiffness. This ratio is an innovative parameter reducing the effects of anatomical differences in different parts of an individual breast. It would, therefore, be possible to compare mechanical parameters of different regions such as medial and lateral parts. Three major states for this ratio were considered as follows:[21]

   - *Ratio≈1*: this means that mechanical properties of the point are very similar to other regions of the breast and usually suggests normal tissue.
   - *Ratio<<1*: this case shows a much softer tissue than the normal texture of the breast. This usually happens in lateral parts of the breast or in the existence of a fatty mass.
   - *Ratio>>1*: this case suggests the existence of a much stiffer tissue than the normal texture of the breast.

Clinical Trial Procedure Robo-Tac-BMI was tested clinically on 161 cases attending a Breast Research Center in Tehran, Iran, in which all patients complained of breast symptoms. According to the Helsinki agreement, the whole study was thoroughly explained to all the patients. Also, in order to have an evaluating criterion, breast sonography, with or without mammography, were chosen as the gold standards. After examination by the system, the results of Robo-Tac-BMI were compared with the other reports. According to the principals of research in medical sciences, to evaluate the accuracy of the Robo-Tac-BMI performance regarding sonography and mammography as the gold standards, the criteria including sensitivity (Sens), specificity (Spec), accuracy (Acc), positive predictive value (PPV), negative predictive value (NPV).[17]

Results The maps of test points of both breasts that were examined by Robo-Tac-BMI are shown in Fig. 9.28. It should be noted that there were symmetrical test points on the maps of both breasts that can be clearly seen. These schematic maps of the scanning test points would be actively provided and contain the information including schematic geometry of the breast tissue, position of the nipple, which is located at the center of the breast, and position of each test points with respect to the nipple. All these test points were defined by two parameters: the angle of each point (which is expressed as the o'clock of that point) and the radius of each point (which is the distance from the nipple).[21]

The force on the horizontal axis against the compression of the tissue on the vertical axis in compression (loading) and relaxation (unloading) processes for two equivalent sample points of breasts of one patient are shown in Fig. 9.29.

Fitting an exponential curve to the output data of the sensors, the graph of Fig. 9.30 would be extracted. It is clear in the graph that there is definitely an abnormal mass in the region of test point 5 which is located at 9 o'clock and also there is a suspicious region in the vicinity of this point which includes test point 6 located at 10 o'clock of the left breast. A simple comparison of loading curves between symmetric points of left and right breasts suggested no suspicious region in the right breast of this patient.

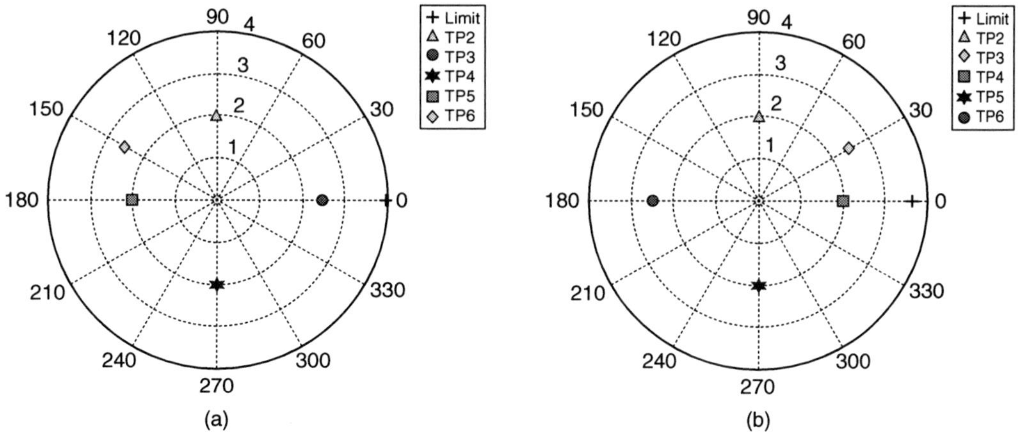

FIGURE 9.28 Schematic map of test points of (*a*) left breast and (*b*) right breast.

A Novel Robotic Tactile Mass Detector with Application in Clinical Breast Examination, Mojra et al., *Minimally Invasive Therapy and Allied Technologies*, In Press, Copyright © [2011], Informa Healthcare. Reproduced with permission of Informa Healthcare.

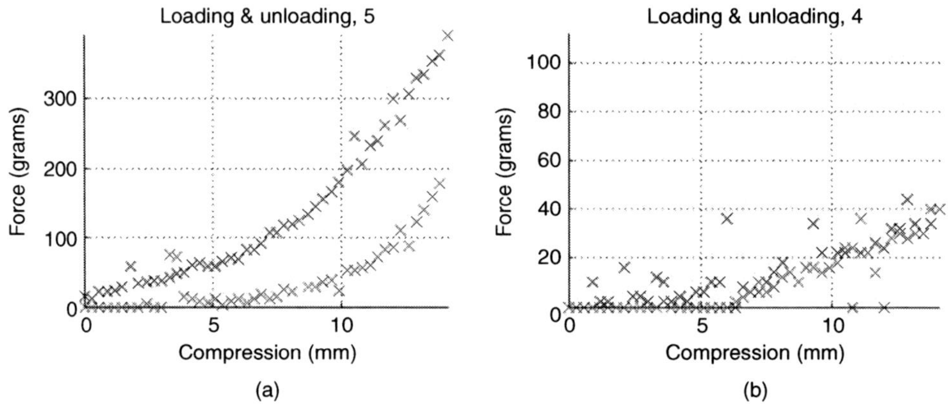

FIGURE 9.29 Active force-displacement diagram in compression (loading) and relaxation (unloading) processes for different test points of (*a*) left breast and (*b*) right breast of a patient. [From Mojra (2011),[18] used by permission.]

The three functional parameters related to the stiffness of the underlying tissue or embedded object is shown in Fig. 9.31. In this figure, each number on the horizontal axis is allocated to a test point on the right breast and the equivalent symmetrical point on the left breast. As can be clearly concluded from the figure, there is a significant difference in *SPS* between 9 o'clock of the left breast and the equivalent point which is 3 o'clock of the right breast. This suggests that there might be a mass near the surface of the breast. Also, there is a marked distinction at the same point of the left breast in *AvS* that confirms the same result. However, there is an apparent increase in *AvS* of point 2 on the left breast, compared to *SPS* of the same point, which is mainly due to the fact that point 2 is in the vicinity of point 3. Finally, from the bar graph showing the *normS,* it can be simply concluded that there are three suspicious points stiffer than the normal tissue:

1. 9 o'clock of the left breast
2. 10 o'clock of the left breast
3. 6 o'clock of the right breast

The exact ratio of measured stiffness parameters are shown in Table 9.7. Suspicious points have clearly a much larger number than the other test points. For the confirmation of the existence of a mass, Mojra et al. suggested that there must be at least two suspicious ratios of three-to-ones to be marked as positive.

Finally, to evaluate the obtained results of Robo-Tac-BMI, breast sonography, with or without mammography, was chosen as the gold standard. After the patients were examined by the robot, the results of Robo-Tac-BMI were compared with the gold standards. For the sample patient, the sonography report contained the following information:[21]

- Normal fibroglandular tissue of the right breast
- No cystic or echodistortion in either breast
- A hypoechoic region at 9 o'clock of the left breast suggestive of a fibroadenoma

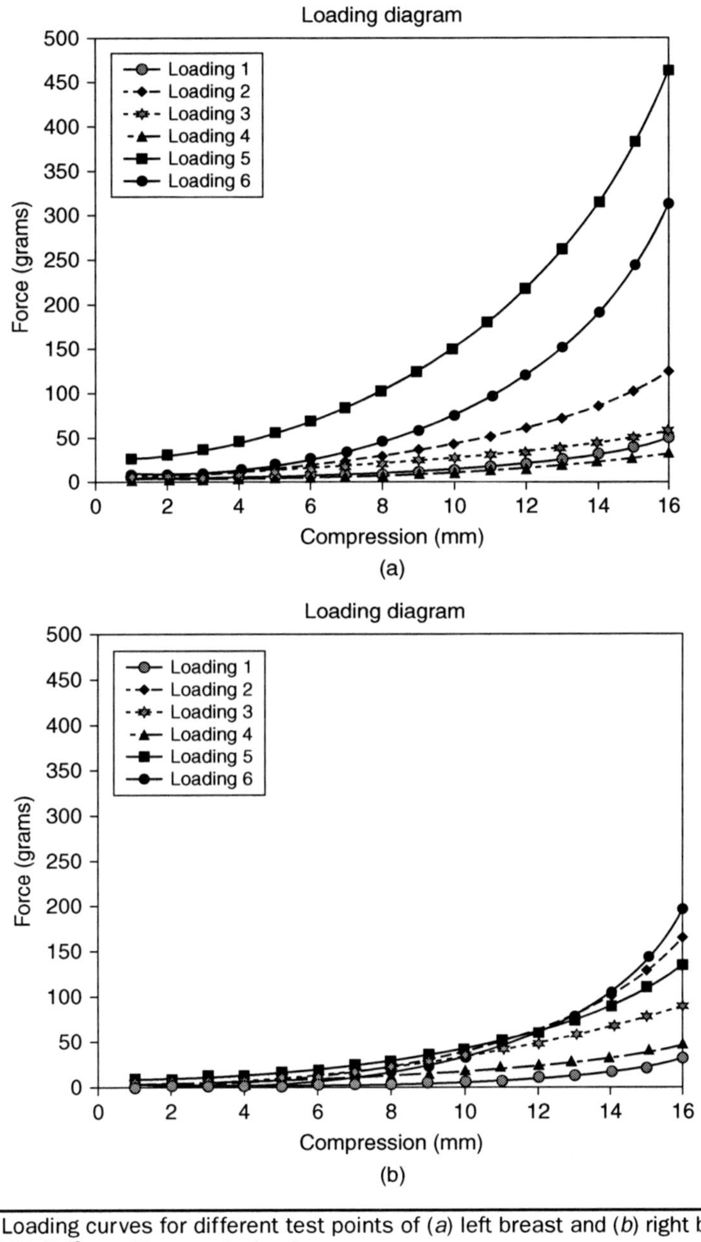

FIGURE 9.30 Loading curves for different test points of (*a*) left breast and (*b*) right breast. [From Mojra (2011),[18] used by permission.]

The mammography report contains the data of increase of breasts' density but there was neither microcalcification nor tissue distortion. According to the gold standards, Mojra et al. concluded that both the sonography and mammography reports evidently confirmed the results of the Robo-Tac-BMI device.

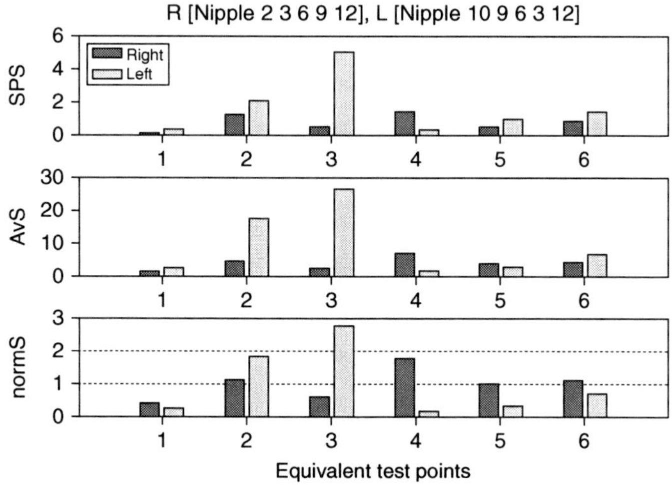

FIGURE 9.31 Three functional stiffness parameters for equivalent symmetric test points on both breasts.

A Novel Robotic Tactile Mass Detector with Application in Clinical Breast Examination, Mojra et al., *Minimally Invasive Therapy and Allied Technologies*, In Press, Copyright © [2011], Informa Healthcare. Reproduced with permission of Informa Healthcare.

	Point Number	**1**	**2**	**3**	**4**	**5**	**6**
Right	O'clock	Nipple	2	3	6	9	12
	SPS_i	0.12	1.32	0.56	1.41	0.58	0.88
	AvS_i	1.73	4.85	2.64	7.52	4.25	4.68
	$normS_i$	0.41	1.13	0.62	1.76	0.99	1.09
Left	O'clock	Nipple	10	9	6	3	12
	SPS_i	0.39	2.08	5.03	0.34	1.04	1.46
	AvS_i	2.77	17.28	26.29	1.74	3.20	6.85
	$normS_i$	0.29	1.78	2.71	0.18	0.33	0.71
Ratio (left/right)	SPS_i	3.38	1.57	8.93	0.24	1.80	1.66
	AvS_i	1.60	3.57	9.96	0.23	0.75	1.46
	$normS_i$	0.70	1.57	4.40	0.10	0.33	0.65

A Novel Robotic Tactile Mass Detector with Application in Clinical Breast Examination, Mojra et al., *Minimally Invasive Therapy and Allied Technologies*, In Press, Copyright © [2011], Informa Healthcare. Reproduced with permission of Informa Healthcare.

TABLE 9.7 Stiffness Parameters Measured for Equivalent Symmetric Test Points on Both Breasts

9.5 Ankle Sprain

One of the most common injuries among athletes is ankle sprain which, especially for football, basketball, and volleyball players, is economically onerous for both the athlete and the organization/s with whom they are affiliated. Ankle sprain occurs when the ankle turns in any direction and places more of a strain on the ligament than it can tolerate. When such an injury occurs, early assessment by a physician is one of the most important factors in order to determine the rest period required and, perhaps even more importantly, when the injury has healed adequately enough for the player to return with no risk of reinjury. Nowadays, doctors usually utilize different imaging technology, such as X-ray or MRI, and move the ankle in different ways to see the status of the injured ligament. Although these methods might be helpful, they only evaluate the ankle when the individual is not subjecting it to any pressure.

Walking is one of the most complex activities that require a very well coordinated use of the neural system and muscles. When one is suffering from ankle sprain, this coordination might change resulting in gait impairment. Analyzing the foot pressure pattern, and investigating abnormalities while walking, is a novel idea that could be used to monitor the status of injured ligaments continually. In the following recently published research work conducted by Nasseri et al.,[24] the above topic has been analyzed using neural networks.

Design and Fabrication of a Novel Insole to Evaluate the Ankle Sprain during the Healing Process A normal gait is symmetrical, which means that gait patterns are similar in both feet.[25–27] By using this fact as a criterion, it is possible to monitor and assess the efficiency of any healing process employed and, ergo, the health status of the athlete. Therefore, when monitoring the gait of an athlete with a sprained ankle during the healing period, and determining the similarities between each foot, it is possible to determine the best time for the athlete to resume their sporting activities. This determination is usually not difficult to make since, due to pain, the athlete cannot distribute his mass equally between his feet and would prefer to place minimum pressure on the injured foot when walking and standing. Supination is another factor that is important in sprained ankle cases. Since ankle sprain may lead to ankle instability, which puts the athlete in danger of recurrent sprains, supination may increase during the stance phase. By analyzing the pressure data on each foot, and extracting these differences, it can be concluded whether or not the sprained ankle has healed adequately.

To accomplish this, a 59-pressure sensor (59PS) system was used to provide essential pressure data for the evaluation of foot pressure in sprained ankle case.[24] The system is a simple, low-cost device designed specifically for evaluating ankle sprains which has the ability to gather only pertinent information for ankle sprain evaluation. Figure 9.32 shows arrangement of the pressure sensors to gather the most important information.

The insole was flexible with a thickness of 0.35 mm. Circular FSRs (force sensitive resistors) having a diameter of 0.35 mm were used as the foot pressure sensors. The size and structure of the system and pressure sensors is shown in Fig. 9.32*a* and *b*. As can be seen in Fig. 9.32*a*, the insole is in the same size as a normal foot. To calibrate the sensors, a force applying mechanism was used. Figure 9.33 shows the calibration system.

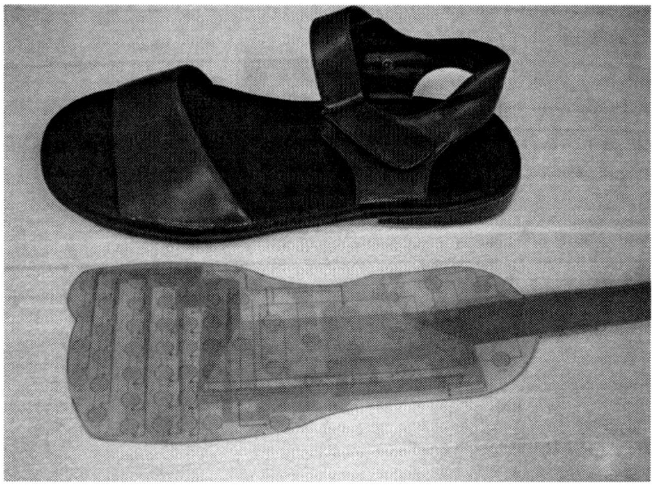

(a)

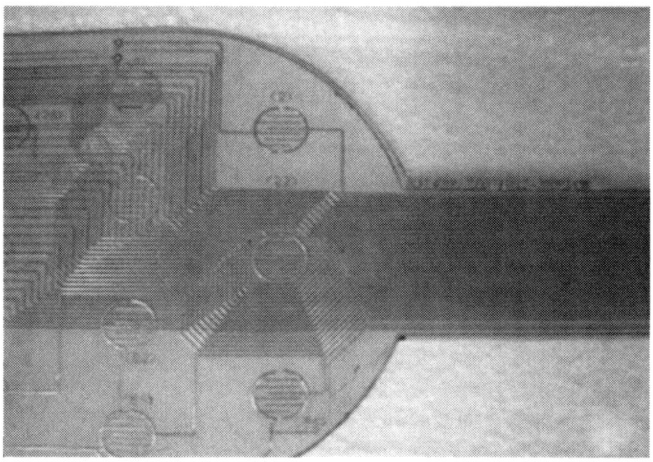

(b)

FIGURE 9.32 (*a*) The insole, and (*b*) A close view of some sensors. [From Nasseri (2009),[28] used by permission.]

Every system that aims to analyze clinical data must include an interface circuit for transmitting data to a computer. A schematic of the interface system used is shown in Fig. 9.34. The circuit consists of four analog multiplexers that are used to transfer data from 64-pressure sensors to the microprocessor. The dimensions of the interface circuit are 9 cm × 5 cm. The outputs from the pressure sensors are collected by a microprocessor unit and are then converted to a 10-bit digital signal (0–1023), at a selected frequency of 100 Hz. Next, the collected data is transmitted through a serial connection to a computer and saved in ".txt" format in the computer. Figure 9.35 shows the final view of the fabricated system.

Segmentation and Feature Extraction A key step in most pattern analysis tasks is feature extraction in which the first step is segmenting the signal. The gait cycle is usually

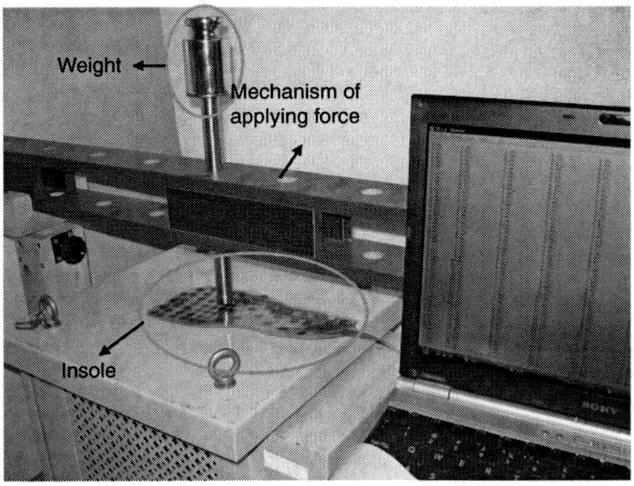

FIGURE 9.33 Calibration system.

A Novel Experimental Analysis for the Scientific Study and Evaluation of Sprained Ankle, Nasseri et al., *Journal of Medical Technology and Physical Therapy*, vol. 23, no. 1, pp. 46–56, 2011. Used by permission.

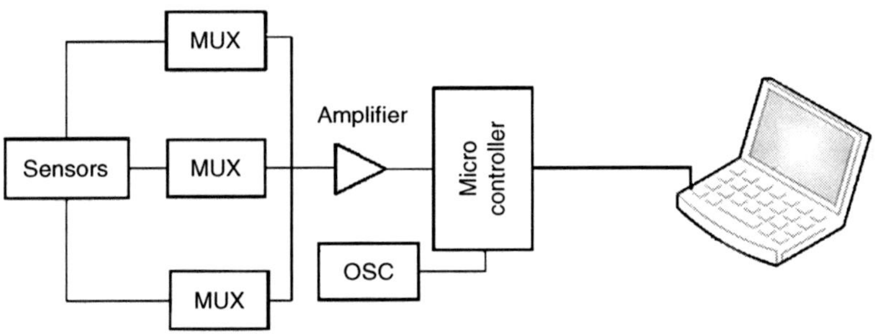

FIGURE 9.34 A schematic of the interface circuit.

"An Embedded Insole, Applicable in Signal Processing: Sprained Ankle Assessment," Nasseri et al., *International Journal of Intelligent Information Technology Application*, vol. 2, no. 4, pp. 144–150, Copyright © 2009. Reproduced with permission of Engineering Technology Press.

divided into different phases and subphases such that each action of the foot and leg can be evaluated at specific sequential time periods. The gait cycle of each leg is divided into the stance phase and the swing phase. The stance phase is the period of time during which the foot is in contact with the ground and the swing phase is the period of time that the foot is off the ground and is swinging forward. In the study conducted by Nasseri et al., segmentation was undertaken in such a way that parts of the gait signal relevant to the stance phase were separated. In this way, a stance phase was detected when more than 80 percent of pressure sensor outputs were on (under pressure).[24] This kind of segmentation could make a large piece of useful information available.

In the next step, to reduce the complexity of classifiers, the most significant features were selected and extracted. Normally, features must be selected in such a way that it can clarify the differences between classes of gait. According to the differences between

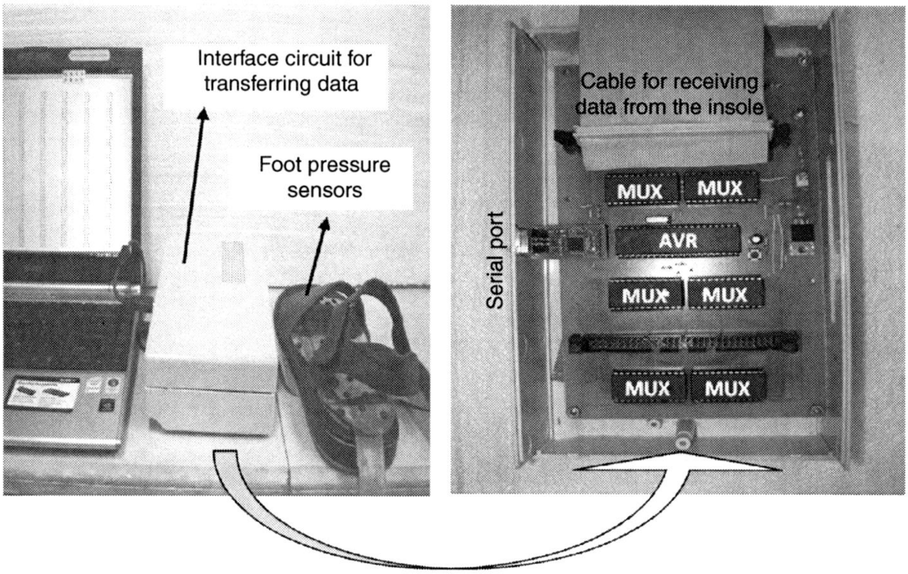

FIGURE 9.35 Final fabricated system.

A Novel Experimental Analysis for the Scientific Study and Evaluation of Sprained Ankle, Nasseri et al., *Journal of Medical Technology and Physical Therapy*, vol. 23, no. 1, pp. 46–56, 2011. Used by permission.

a normal gait and the gait of an athlete with a sprained ankle, four features of gait signal were selected: maximum force on each foot during the stance phase, stance phase duration, swing phase duration, and supination during stance phase.

Also, there must be a classifier to classify the wide range of gathered data. The most widely used classifiers are the artificial neural networks (ANNs), support vector machines, k-nearest neighbors, Gaussian mixture model, Gaussian, naive bayes, decision tree, and RBF classifiers. As discussed in Chap. 6, the greatest advantage of ANNs is their ability to "learn" from observed data. However, using them is not so straightforward and a relatively good understanding of the underlying theory is essential.

Multilayer perceptrons (MLPs) are able to represent the most prominent and well-researched class of ANNs in classification, implementing a feed forward, supervised and hetero-associative paradigm. MLPs with at least three layers would be capable of approximating any desired bounded continuous function.

To classify the normal and sprained ankle plantar pressure patterns, the MLP algorithm was used. The specified neural network, having the typical feed forward structure with one hidden layer as shown in Fig. 9.36, is based on the back propagation supervised learning algorithm. The multilayer structure allows the neural network to capture the internal representations of rather complex input patterns by the development of internal representations.[30] To provide an efficient way of implementing the gradient descent method for such a multilayered network, the back propagation algorithm (delta rule) was applied.

The work and efficiency of this suggested classification procedure was tested by a set of simulated data. In this way, the neural network was trained using a set of labeled simulated plantar pressure data.

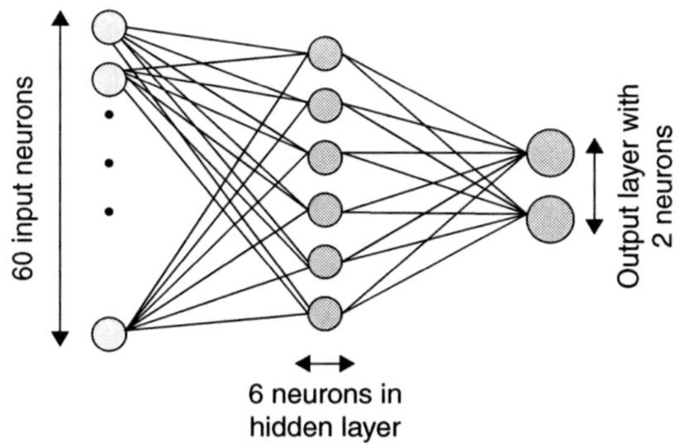

FIGURE 9.36 Feed forward neural network with one hidden layer.
"An Embedded Insole, Applicable in Signal Processing: Sprained Ankle Assessment," Nasseri et al., *International Journal of Intelligent Information Technology Application*, vol. 2, no. 4, pp. 144–150, Copyright © 2009. Reproduced with permission of Engineering Technology Press.

Plantar pressure distribution of 70 persons from two groups of normal and sprained ankle athletes was selected as the training data and the plantar pressure distribution of thirty persons in each group was selected as the testing data. The training phase consisted of the following steps:[29]

1. Set all network weights to random values between – 1 and + 1.
2. Select a training set of examples from both the healthy and sprained ankle group.
3. Determine the network output (normal or sprained ankle).
4. Compare the output of the network to the desired values.
5. Determine the "error" associated with each neuron, typically based on the difference between the desired and actual outputs.
6. Adjust the weight matrix for the neurons based on the "error."
7. Select a different input from the input set.
8. If all the input data have been presented to the network, go to step 9, otherwise repeat steps 2 to 8.
9. Determine whether all "errors" are within an acceptable range.
10. If "errors" are unacceptable, repeat steps 3 to 4.

One of the main features of a neural network algorithm is that it has the ability to generalize by correctly classifying unknown data. Since there is no guarantee that the network could achieve the desired characteristics of generalization at the termination of the training phase, a testing phase was required to determine if this had been learned by the network during training. The testing of the network proceeded in the following manner:[29]

1. Select test data from the test set and apply it to the previously trained network.
2. Determine if the desired outputs of the network and the actual outputs match within some tolerance.

3. If the outputs do not match, then the plantar pressure pattern has been incorrectly classified. If a match does occur, then the plantar pressure pattern has been correctly classified.
4. If the error of classification is more than the desired expectation, the iterations of the training phase will increase and the error of the training phase will be decreased. Step 1 through step 3 will be repeated. Step 4 will be repeated until the network has demonstrated sufficient ability to classify (e.g., a specific percentage of tests are correctly classified).

Also, it should be considered that ankle sprains usually occur when the ankle supination is more than a defined threshold. The regression model is shown as Eq. (9.1),[31] with SupT, as the supination torque of the foot, in N-m, and P_X as the value of pressure of the sensor at position x, in N/cm^2:

$$\text{SupT}(N.m) = -2.068 + 0.910 \times (P_{60}) + 1.318 \times (P_{72}) + 1.549 \times (P_{98}) + \text{error} \tag{9.1}$$

where P_{60}, P_{72}, and P_{98} are the three pressure data that are essential to reconstruct the ankle supination torque.[31]

As previously mentioned, one big problem with having a sprained ankle is that it could lead to ankle instability and increased ankle supination during daily activities. This means that the essential differences between the pressure distribution patterns of a normal foot, compared to an ankle-sprained foot during walking, are in the magnitudes of pressure in the three specified points.

To simulate the plantar pressure of healthy and sprained ankle cases, 200 matrices were generated during walking; 100 for healthy and 100 for ankle sprained cases.[31] The magnitude of plantar pressure in three specified regions in the ankle sprained group was greater than the magnitude of pressure in the same regions in the normal group. Figure 9.37 shows the difference, during walking, between the plantar pressure pattern of a sample simulated normal foot and a sample simulated ankle sprained foot.

The network was started with a training set of 140 patterns. Figure 9.38 shows the network error against the iterations of network training in which it can be seen that the total error of the network during the training phase decreases in proportion to the increase in the iteration of network training. To evaluate the learning classification abilities of the developed network, a test set of 60 plantar pressure patterns was used of which none was present in the training set.

The percentage of correctly classified plantar pressure patterns is shown in Table 9.8. It can be observed that the network is significantly able to generalize the data.

To determine whether or not the system can help to distinguish between a healthy ankle and a sprained ankle, experimental studies were performed on six male athletes in whom it had been determined that their natural tendency was to place more weight on their left foot. Their ages ranged between 17 ± 5 years, height = 1.85 ± 0.05 m, body mass = 85 ± 10 kg, foot length = 244 to 245 mm).[24] They were asked to wear sandals, in which one sandal had a pressure measurement insole embedded. Participants performed two trials of walking in a clinic, ten steps in each trial. Three of the participants suffered from left-ankle sprain but had a normal right foot. The other three were normal athletes with no disorder in either of their lower limbs or feet and were taken as the control group.

The following four features were taken as being the main criteria from which to extract comparative data, namely: maximum force on the foot (N), stance phase

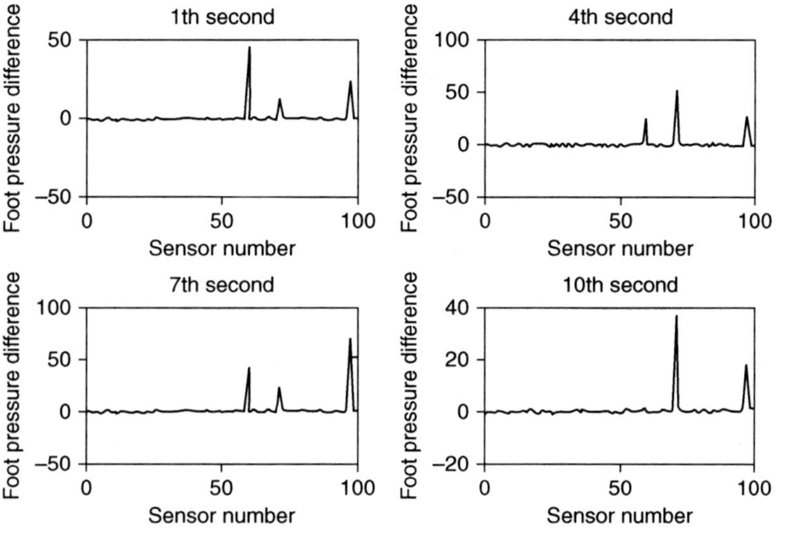

Figure 9.37 The difference, during walking, between the plantar pressure pattern of a simulated normal foot and a simulated ankle sprained foot.

"An Embedded Insole, Applicable in Signal Processing: Sprained Ankle Assessment," Nasseri et al., *International Journal of Intelligent Information Technology Application*, vol. 2, no. 4, pp. 144–150, Copyright © 2009. Reproduced with permission of Engineering Technology Press.

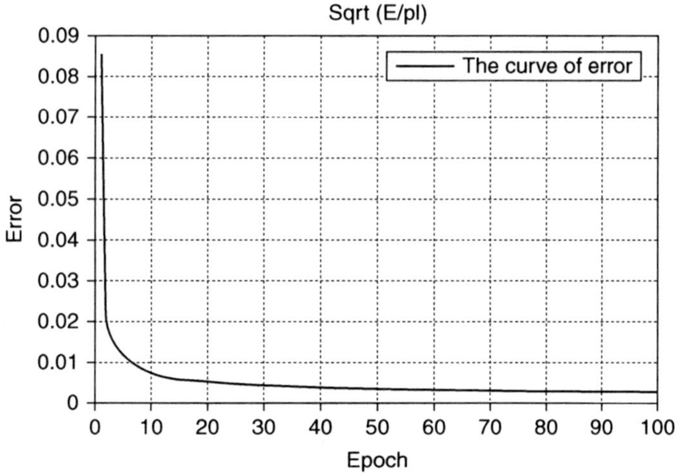

Figure 9.38 Network error against the iterations of network training.

"An Embedded Insole, Applicable in Signal Processing: Sprained Ankle Assessment," Nasseri et al., *International Journal of Intelligent Information Technology Application*, vol. 2, no. 4, pp. 144–150, Copyright © 2009. Reproduced with permission of Engineering Technology Press.

The Accuracy of Classifying in Training Phase		The Accuracy of Classifying in Testing Phase	
Total accuracy of classifying: 99%		Total accuracy of classifying: 97.9%	
Accuracy of normal pattern recognition:	Accuracy of sprained ankle pattern recognition:	Accuracy of normal pattern recognition:	Accuracy of sprained ankle pattern recognition:
98%	99%	97.5%	98%

"An Embedded Insole, Applicable in Signal Processing: Sprained Ankle Assessment," Nasseri et al., *International Journal of Intelligent Information Technology Application*, vol. 2, no. 4, pp. 144–150, Copyright © 2009. Reproduced with permission of Engineering Technology Press.

TABLE 9.8 The Percentage of Plantar Pressure Patterns That Were Classified Correctly

duration (S), swing phase duration (S), and supination (N-m), where N is newton, N-m is newton-meters, and S is seconds.

Results In order to evaluate the status of an athlete after ankle sprain, data from the above four features were extracted and significant differences were seen between the control group and the group with a sprained ankle. Figure 9.39 shows the readings in an athlete having a strained left ankle. Figure 9.40 shows the readings of each of the three athletes with a sprained ankle and Fig. 9.41 shows the readings of one of the normal athletes in the control group. In Fig. 9.40, it can be seen that there is a significant difference in magnitude of readings for each of the three athletes with a sprained ankle whereas, as shown in Fig. 9.41, for a normal athlete these readings are virtually identical in each foot.

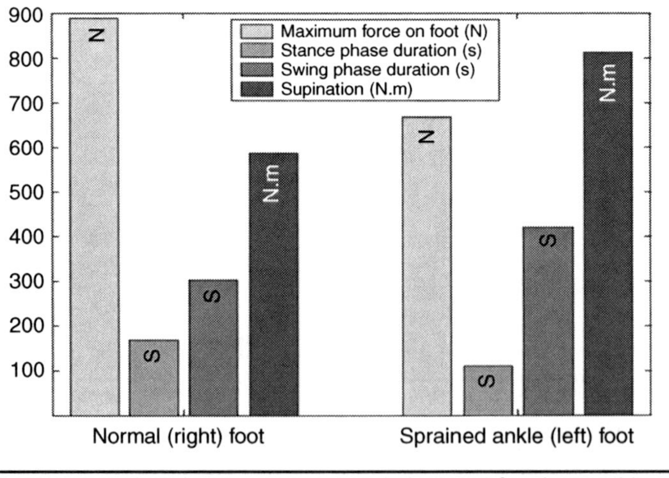

FIGURE 9.39 Feature comparison between normal and abnormal foot in an athlete with sprained ankle.

A Novel Experimental Analysis for the Scientific Study and Evaluation of Sprained Ankle, Nasseri et al., *Journal of Medical Technology and Physical Therapy*, vol. 23, no. 1, pp. 46–56, 2011. Used by permission.

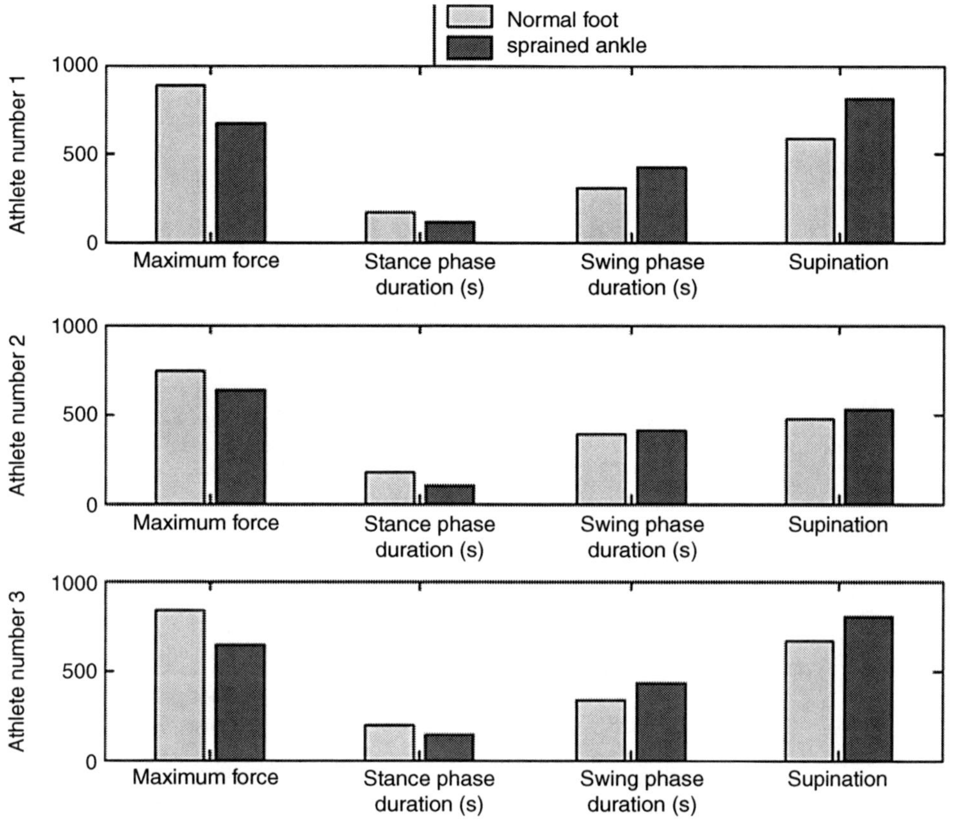

FIGURE 9.40 Differences in extracted features for each volunteer athlete.

A Novel Experimental Analysis for the Scientific Study and Evaluation of Sprained Ankle, Nasseri et al., *Journal of Medical Technology and Physical Therapy*, vol. 23, no. 1, pp. 46–56, 2011. Used by permission.

As can be seen from Fig. 9.40, the difference in duration of the stance phase and swing phase of the sprained ankle is markedly evident whereas in a normal athlete, as shown in Fig. 9.41, there is very little difference. It can also be seen that, for each of the three athletes in Fig. 9.40, supination in the sprained ankle increases compared to the normal foot. However, the same difference also occurs in a normal case as shown in Fig. 9.41 so it is possible that this difference could also be attributable to other factors such as bad walking habits.

Differences between magnitudes of each feature in the group with a sprained ankle, in comparison to the control group, are shown in Tables 9.9 and 9.10.

It can easily be seen during the stance phase that the athlete with a sprained ankle will naturally wish to transfer as much force as possible from his sprained ankle onto his normal foot in order to alleviate his pain and discomfort.[24]

Also, a comparison between the supination magnitude in Tables 9.9 and 9.10 demonstrates that although this feature is larger in a sprained ankle in comparison with a normal foot, other factors are also responsible for increasing supination, such as bad walking habits, etc. Increased supination may also occur in a normal case so it should not, therefore, be considered as a comparison factor in evaluating sprained ankles.[24]

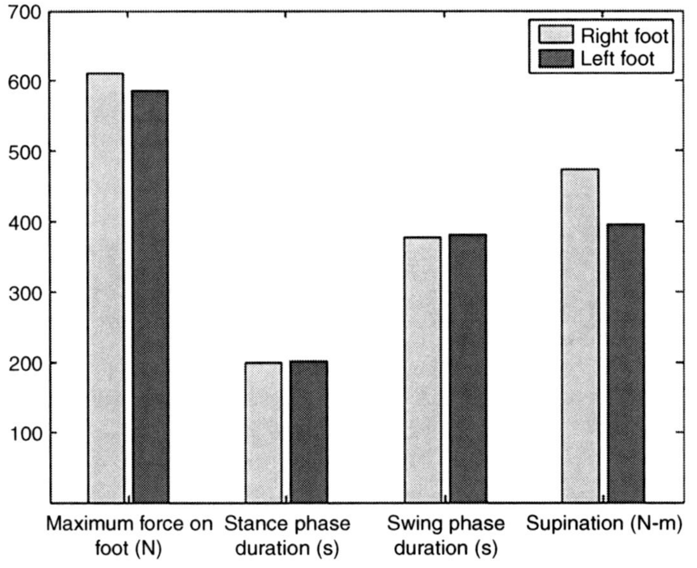

Figure 9.41 Feature comparison between feet of a volunteer normal athlete.
A Novel Experimental Analysis for the Scientific Study and Evaluation of Sprained Ankle, Nasseri et al., *Journal of Medical Technology and Physical Therapy*, vol. 23, no. 1, pp. 46–56, 2011. Used by permission.

Foot	Whole Force (N)	Mid-Stance Duration (S)	Swing Duration (S)	Supination (N-m)
Right	888	0.3361	0.6037	29.3210
Left (Sprained)	668	0.2193	0.8401	40.6462
Difference between the two feet%	−32.93%	−53.26%	28.14%	27.86%

A Novel Experimental Analysis for the Scientific Study and Evaluation of Sprained Ankle, Nasseri et al., *Journal of Medical Technology and Physical Therapy*, vol. 23, no. 1, pp. 46–56, 2011. Used by permission.

Table 9.9 Magnitude of Each Feature in an Athlete in the Group with Sprained Ankle

Foot	Whole Force (N)	Mid-Stance Duration (S)	Swing Duration (S)	Supination (N-m)
Right	611	0.3990	0.7556	23.6806
Left (Sprained)	587	0.4041	0.7621	19.8212
Difference between the two feet (%)	−4.09%	1.26%	0.85%	−19.47%

A Novel Experimental Analysis for the Scientific Study and Evaluation of Sprained Ankle, Nasseri et al., *Journal of Medical Technology and Physical Therapy*, vol. 23, no. 1, pp. 46–56, 2011. Used by permission.

Table 9.10 Magnitude of Each Feature in an Athlete in the Control Group

9.6 Active Prosthetic Knee

Amputation of the lower extremity is one of the main sources of disability that affects individuals' lives. In the United States, it has been estimated that 1.9 million people have lost a limb, of whom 400,000 have had amputations above the knee.[32] For these people, a prosthetic leg that includes a socket, knee, shank, and foot is usually prescribed. Despite the fact that there have been significant advances in the design and fabrication of these different parts, one of the main problems with currently available prosthetic knees is that they are unable to generate enough net power and hence are too passive. A prosthetic knee needs to be active in generating net power because a patient who has undergone a transfemoral amputation consumes a lot more energy than a normal person,[33] and exerts a torque on his/her hip that is three times larger than normal.[34]

The lower the level of amputation, however, the better the gait performance will be by the amputee.[35] The reason for this, as previously mentioned, is that during the middle stance phase of gait, a normal knee enables the person to move forward on his/her single flexed knee by generating power. Due to the fact that currently available commercial prosthetic knees are not capable of generating sufficient net power, the patient needs to consume more energy in order to move forward on one single extended knee. A study conducted by Dabiri et al.[36] compared the flexion angle of an active and passive knee joint with a biologically normal knee. They considered two models of the lower extremity in which each was modeled as a two-DOF pendulum, one for the hip and another for the knee joint. Using MSC ADAMS software, a passive prosthetic knee was modeled that used a hinge joint with a damper and a spring (Fig. 9.42). Using MATLAB

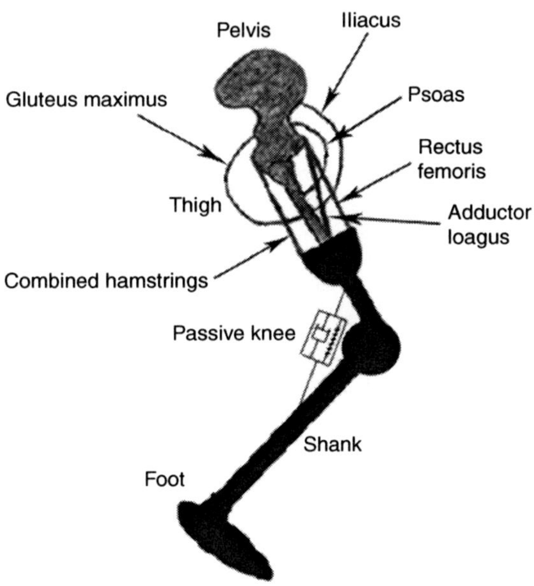

FIGURE 9.42 Schematic of the lower extremity with a passive prosthetic knee.

Dabiri et al., "Comparison of Passive and Active Prosthetic Knee Joint Kinematics during Swing Phase of Gait," Proceedings of 17th Iranian Conference on Biomedical Engineering (ICBME 2010), Isfahan, Iran, November 2010, © IEEE.

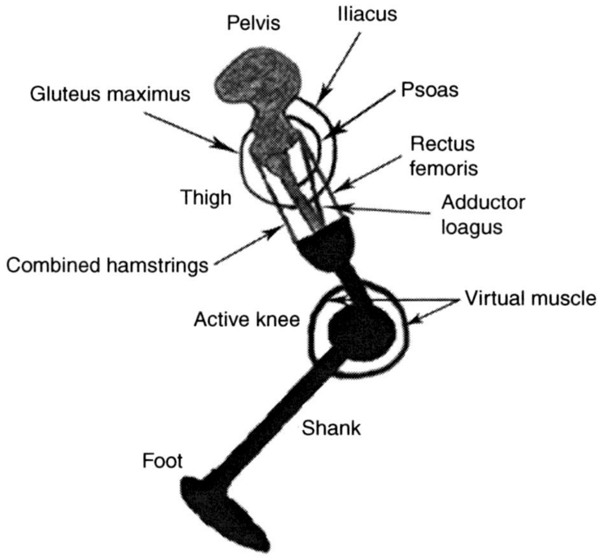

FIGURE 9.43 Schematic of the prosthetic leg with an active prosthetic knee. The knee has a pair of antagonist muscles that deliver power.

Dabiri et al., "Comparison of Passive and Active Prosthetic Knee Joint Kinematics during Swing Phase of Gait," Proceedings of 17th Iranian Conference on Biomedical Engineering (ICBME 2010), Isfahan, Iran, November 2010, © IEEE.

software, an active prosthetic knee was modeled which included a pair of virtual antagonist muscles (Fig. 9.43).

The inputs of the models were considered to be normal hip and knee angles,[37] and the torque at these joints were calculated in such a way that the desired input angles were produced. Calculation of the values of stiffness and damping coefficient of the knee in the first model was achieved by an optimization analysis using the least square method. In the second model, to produce the desired knee angle, the forces of the antagonist muscles must have already been calculated.[38] The governing equation of the models is shown as follows in Eq. (9.2):[39]

$$\begin{bmatrix} \ddot{\theta}_H \\ -\ddot{\theta}_K \end{bmatrix} = M^{-1}C\begin{bmatrix} \dot{\theta}_H^2 \\ \dot{\theta}_K^2 \end{bmatrix} + M^{-1}V\begin{bmatrix} -\dot{\theta}_H\dot{\theta}_K \\ 0.0 \end{bmatrix} + M^{-1}G + M^{-1}\begin{bmatrix} M_H \\ -M_K \end{bmatrix} \tag{9.2}$$

where $\ddot{\theta}_H$ and $\ddot{\theta}_K$ are hip and shank rotational accelerations, respectively. M, C, V, and G depend upon joint angles and inertial parameters. M_H is the torque resulting from the muscle forces about the hip joint, and M_K is the torque about the knee joint. In the passive model, M_K is produced by the damper and spring forces, and in the active model it results from the virtual muscles activation that span the knee.

The knee angle during the swing phase of a gait cycle for active and passive prosthetic joints, and a biological knee is shown in Fig. 9.44. As can be seen in the figure, an active prosthetic knee joint can track the biological knee angle much better than a passive prosthetic knee, although the passive knee flexion angle is closer to the biological one.

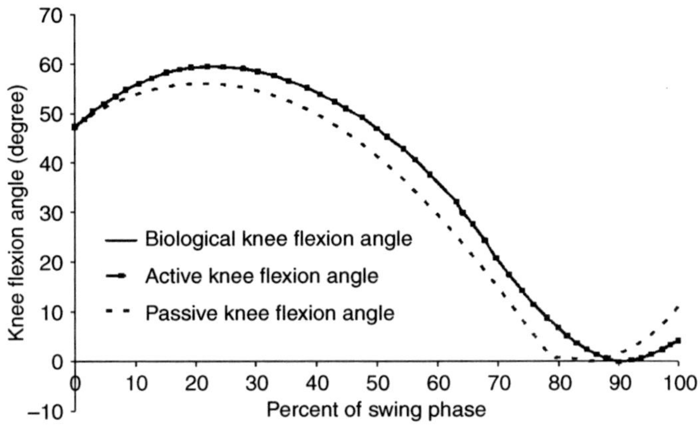

FIGURE 9.44 Biological (desired), active, and passive knee flexion angles, during swing phase. Dabiri et al., "Comparison of Passive and Active Prosthetic Knee Joint Kinematics during Swing Phase of Gait," Proceedings of 17th Iranian Conference on Biomedical Engineering (ICBME 2010), Isfahan, Iran, November 2010, © IEEE.

As a result, it was concluded that although a passive prosthetic knee joint can produce a knee flexion angle nearer to that of a normal one, a powered prosthetic knee is capable of emulating the biological knee angle much better than a passive one.

The above discussion may show why a thorough study of the research topic into the design and fabrication of active, power generator knees has been kept in abeyance for so long.

In 2008, Sup et al.[40] developed an active prosthetic foot including an active ankle and knee that was equipped with pneumatic actuators. Using an impedance control, they could control the torque exerted on the ankle and knee joint in such a way that it simulates the torque exerted on a normal ankle and knee joint. The impedance control is used to divide a gait cycle into different modes during each of which different parameters are controlled in such a way that the generated torque is similar to that exerted on a normal ankle or knee. To bring the amount of torque τ exerted on the prosthetic ankle and knee into agreement with a biological foot, Sup et al. employed Eq. (9.3) as follows:[40, 34]

$$\tau = k_1(\theta - \theta_e) + k_2(\theta - \theta_e)^3 + b\dot{\theta} \tag{9.3}$$

where θ_e is the balance angle, θ is the angle of ankle or knee, k_1 is the linear coefficient, k_2 is the cubic coefficient, b is the linear damping coefficient of the system.

In 2010, Dabiri et al.[43] calculated the required force that needed to be generated in artificial flexor and extensor muscles so that the torque in the hip and knee are the same as a normal biological hip and knee.

For muscles to control the motion of hip and knee joints, the following equality constraint must be valid as shown in Eq. (9.4):[37]

$$\begin{bmatrix} \ddot{\tau}_H \\ \ddot{\tau}_K \end{bmatrix} - \begin{bmatrix} (\ddot{\tau}_H)_{\text{exp.}} \\ (\ddot{\tau}_K)_{\text{exp.}} \end{bmatrix} = 0.0 \tag{9.4}$$

where $(\ddot{\tau}_H)_{exp}$, and $(\ddot{\tau}_K)_{exp}$ are the experimental calculated torque at the hip and knee joints respectively. The amounts of $\ddot{\tau}_H$ and $\ddot{\tau}_K$ are calculated by multiplying the force generated in each muscle by its moment arm. Since it can be assumed that during normal walking each muscle acts like an ideal force generator, then each muscle's force could be calculated by using Eq. (9.5):[41]

$$F = aF_{max} \tag{9.5}$$

where a is the value of muscle activations between 0 and 1.0, F_{max} is the maximum isometric force generated in a muscle and F is the muscle's force. The moment arm of each muscle is calculated by Eq. (9.6):[42]

$$ma = (\partial l^{MT} / \partial q_i) \tag{9.6}$$

where l^{MT} is the total length of the actuators and q_i is the symbol of the axis with what the torque is considered to have in the same direction. Since the number of unknowns (muscle forces) is too numerous, an optimization approach through minimum normal stress of muscles was used as described in Eq. (9.7):[41]

$$J = \sum_{m=1}^{MN} (a_m)^2 \tag{9.7}$$

where J is the optimization parameter, MN is the number of muscles, and a_m is a constant that is multiplied in each muscle's maximum force. Figure 9.45 shows the amount of calculated force generated by the artificial flexor and extensor muscles.

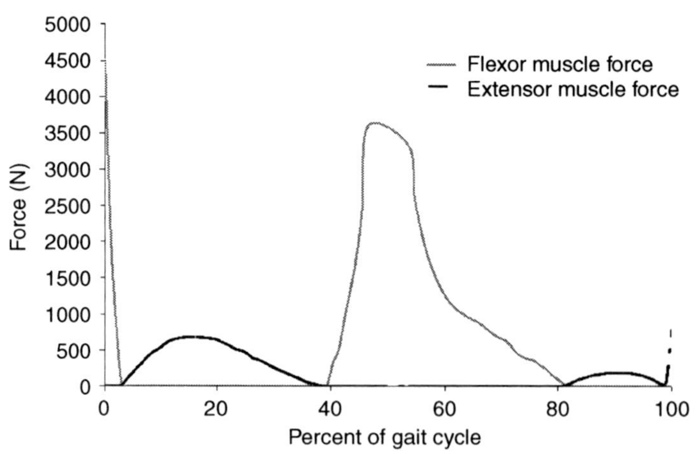

FIGURE 9.45 Calculated forces of artificial flexor and extensor muscles. [From Dabiri (2010),[43] used by permission.]

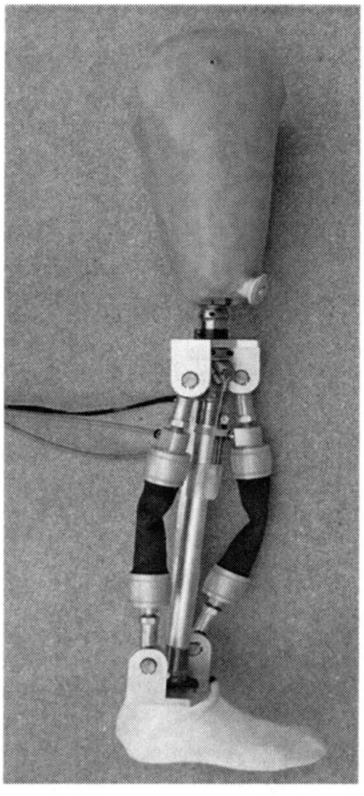

FIGURE 9.46 The view of an active prosthetic knee joint. [From Dabiri (2010),[43] used by permission.]

In Fig. 9.46, a view of the active knee joint designed and fabricated by Dabiri et al.[43] is shown. To control the joint, i.e. the activation algorithm of the artificial muscles, a gait cycle was divided into different modes as shown in Fig. 9.47. In each mode, the muscles are activated in such a way that the knee angle is as similar as possible to a normal one. To determine the mode of gait cycle, two on/off sensors, as shown in Fig. 9.48, were installed at the sole of the foot that could detect the contact of heel and paw. An angular potentiometer was also used to determine the knee angle. Data from the sensors were transferred to a computer using a data accusation card and were processed by the LABVIEW program. Finally, the program would determine the amount of input pressure to the artificial muscles according to the mode of gait.

The fabricated prosthetic knee was tested clinically, while the motion of ankle, knee, and hip joint were tracked using three markers and high-speed cameras. Figure 9.49 shows different modes of gait and Fig. 9.50 shows the angle of the prosthetic knee during one single cycle of gait. The active prosthetic knee can track the normal biological knee angle which verified the fact that the prosthetic knee was able to flex the knee during the stance phase of gait. It should be noted that a passive prosthetic knee normally makes the patient, who has had a transfemoral amputation, unable to flex the knee during the stance so, therefore, the prosthetic joint remains stable,[44] causing more consumption of energy. The power at the prosthetic knee is calculated using the torque and angle of the knee during a cycle of gait and is shown in Fig. 9.51. Since

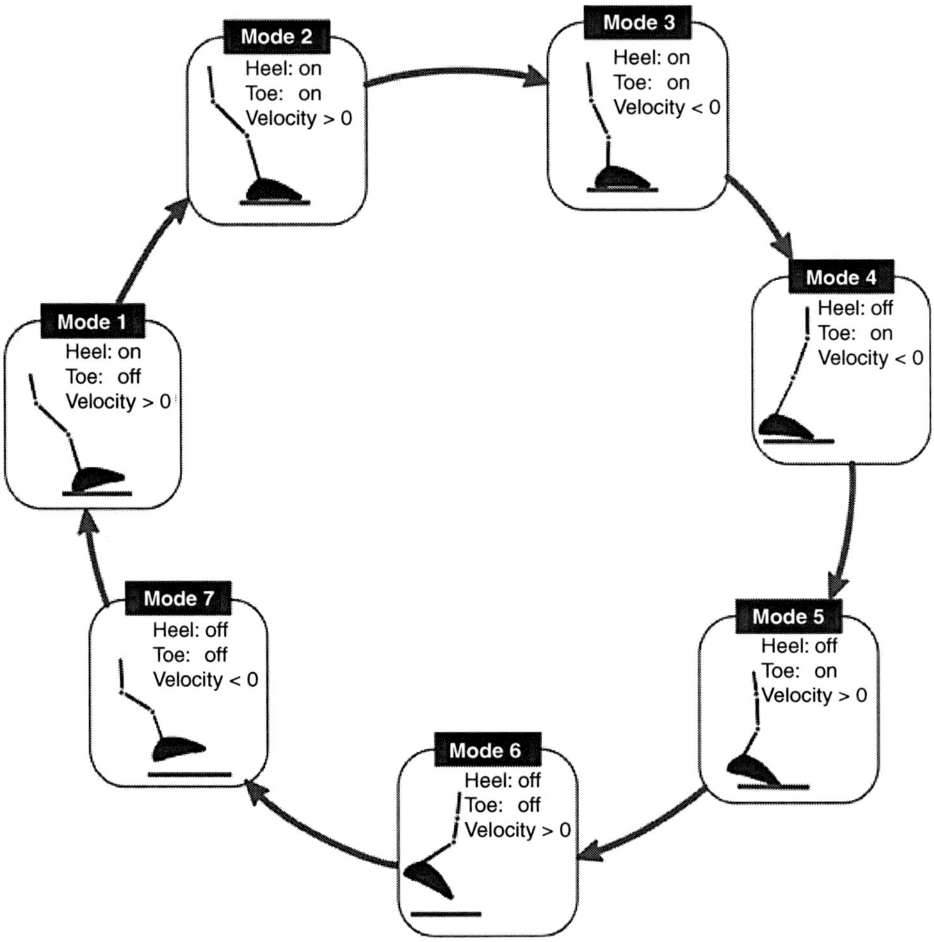

Figure 9.47 Different modes of a normal gait cycle. [From Dabiri (2010),[43] used by permission.]

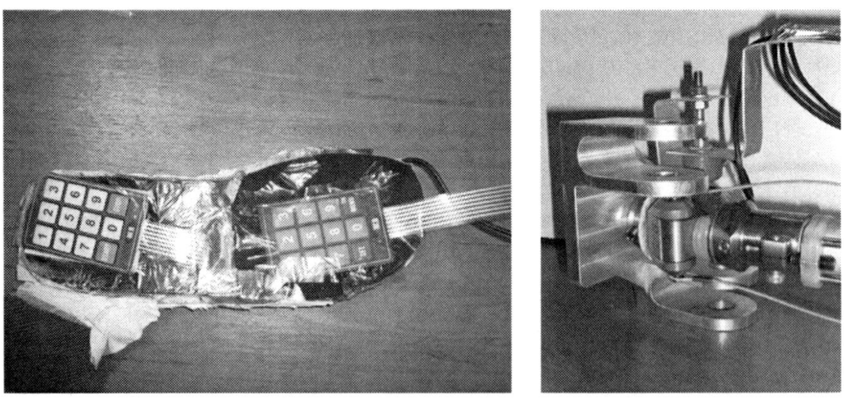

(a) (b)

Figure 9.48 (*a*) On/off sensors, and (*b*) The angular potentiometer used to determine the mode of gait. [From Dabiri (2010),[43] used by permission.]

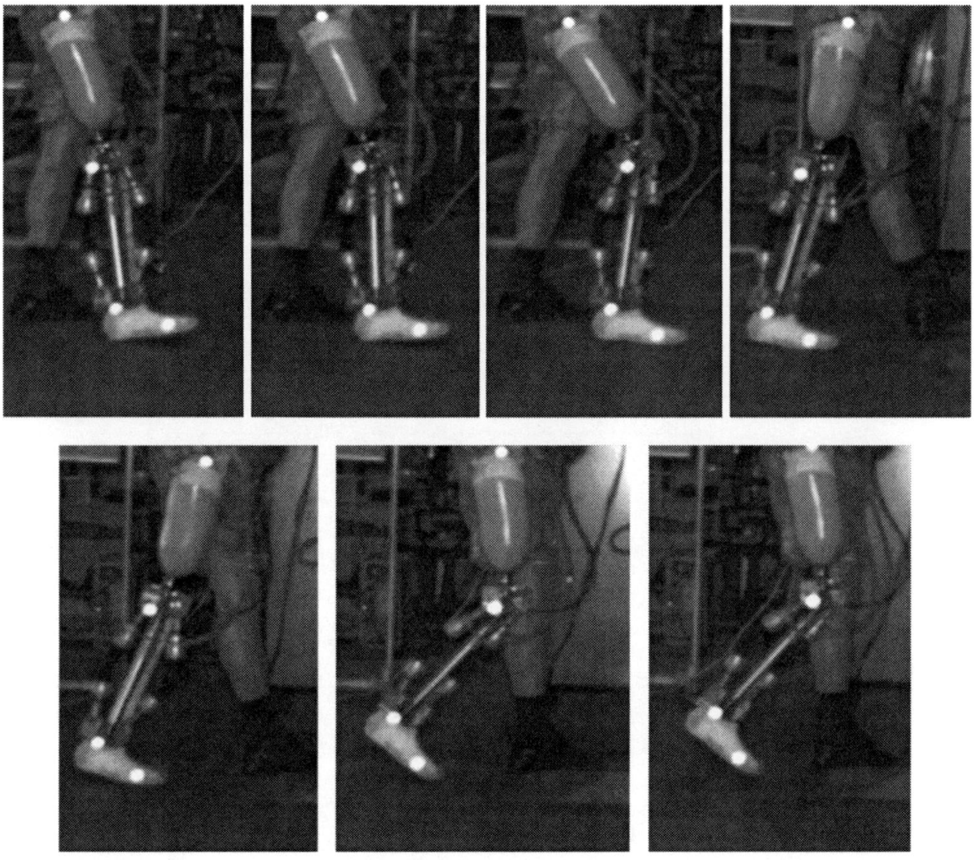

FIGURE 9.49 A sequence of different modes of gait. [From Dabiri (2010),[43] used by permission.]

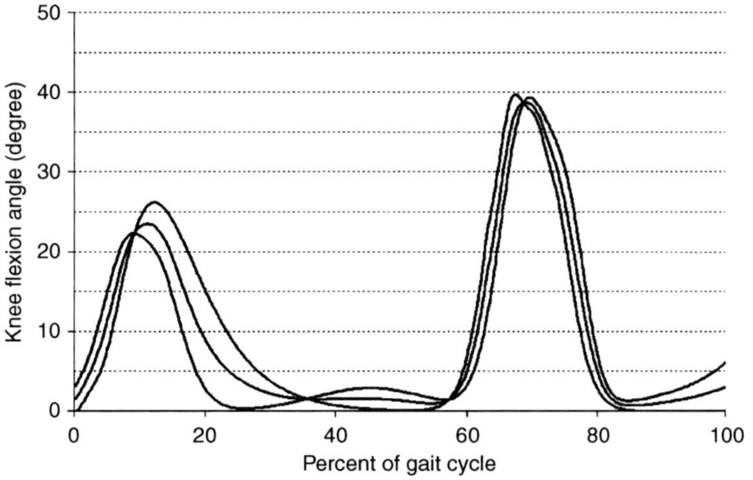

FIGURE 9.50 Angle of prosthetic knee during a cycle of gait during the experiment. [From Dabiri (2010),[43] used by permission.]

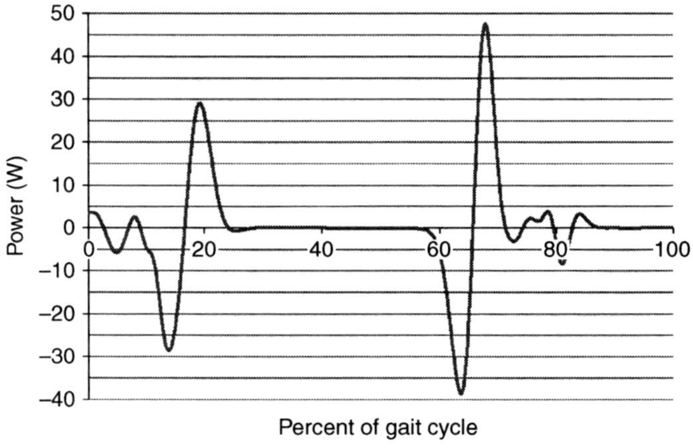

FIGURE 9.51 Power of the prosthetic knee during a cycle of gait. [From Dabiri (2010),[43] used by permission.]

transferring this significant amount of power produced an angle similar to that of a normal knee, it was concluded that using an active prosthetic knee can help the amputee to walk more smoothly and easily.

9.7 Smart System for Cardiovascular Plaque Detection

Distinguishing between different tissues and organs during open surgery is mainly achieved by the surgeon's sense of touch. The surgeon also, by determining the force required, is usually able to prevent damage and injury.[16] One of the main tasks when application of this sense is most critical is when the surgeon is required to cut tissue close to an artery. In such cases, the surgeon usually touches and palpates the surface of the tissue to detect for a pulse which is indicative of the presence of an artery. However, it is not unknown for an artery to be cut accidentally during surgery either due to the surgeon making a sense of touch error or the blood pulse was dampened because of atherosclerosis. The problem becomes even more compounded during minimally invasive laparoscopic surgery when the surgeon may require to accesses internal tissues and organs through four or five incisions. In this type of surgery, which is becoming very popular, the surgeon does not touch the tissues directly but views the procedure indirectly on a 2D monitor screen. Because laparoscopic surgery utilizes slender instruments, the incision is either cauterized to reduce the amount of blood or grippers are placed on either side.[45] However, to assist the surgeon in detecting and locating the presence of either a small or stenotic artery, more research is required. Some solutions have been suggested; nearly all based on imaging and ultrasound approaches. Although these methods might be helpful at some levels, incorrect results can occur for the same reasons as when a surgeon fails to detect an artery during open surgery thereby highlighting the necessity of developing a more reliable approach.

Experimental and Numerical Analysis of Tactile Detection and Examination of Arteries Artificial tactile sensing is a new technique for detecting of arteries in soft tissues by

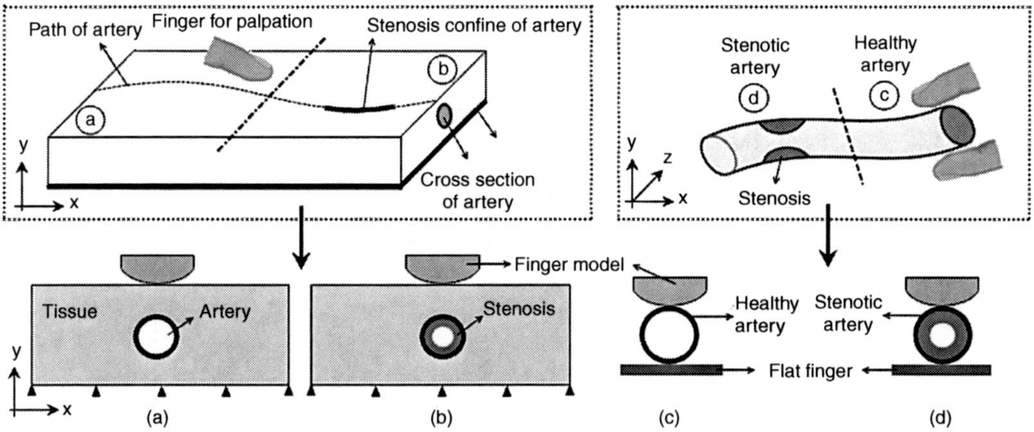

Figure 9.52 Schematic representations of four models. (*a*) Tissue including a healthy artery. (*b*) Tissue including a stenotic artery. (*c*) Healthy artery out of tissue. (*d*) Stenotic artery out of tissue.

Abouei et al., "A Novel Method in Exploration of Arteries Inside a Tissue and Assessment of the Arteries by Computational Approach," Proceedings of the IEEE/ASME International Conference on Advanced Intelligent Mechatronics (AIM), Montreal, Canada, July 2010, © IEEE.

palpation.[46,47] Recently, a novel, tactile sensing based method was proposed and modeled by Abouei et al. that not only can detect the presence of an artery, but also can diagnose whether the artery suffers from atherosclerosis.[48]

Numerical Modeling The technique generally used in tactile detection of an artery is to palpate the tissues and extract the contact data as shown in Fig. 9.52. To determine whether or not the proposed technique could distinguish a healthy artery from a stenotic artery, different models, such as that shown in Fig. 9.52, were developed and stress graphs were extracted of the tissue surface where the contact occurs. The cross-section of the parts pass in the x-y plane through the center of the healthy artery and the stenotic artery.

In the modeling, the arteries were assumed to be completely circular with a diameter of 2.25 mm and mean wall thickness of 0.315 mm. The centers of the arteries were assumed to be at a distance of 10 mm from the top side and 30 mm from the left and the right sides of the models. The soft tissue and the arteries were considered to be elastic and isotropic.[49] The blood pressure waveform of the brachial artery, was applied into the inside wall of the arteries for simulating the effect of blood on the artery wall.[49,50]

Effect of Rolling During vascular surgery, it is a very common for the surgeon to roll the artery extracted from adjacent tissues to determine the exact location of the stenosis and whether or not he/she is dealing with an axisymmetric or non-axisymmetric plaque. To analyze this, three different arteries, including a healthy artery, an axisymmetric stenotic artery, and a non-axisymmetric stenotic artery were modeled. A supposition vertical line stick to models *b* and *c* was considered and then, for every step of solution, the arteries were rotated 45 degrees until a 360-degree rotation is completed. Half of this rolling procedure is illustrated in Fig. 9.53.

Results As previously mentioned, contact data needed to be extracted from the surface of the tissues. As a result, the von Mises stress values were extracted from the top

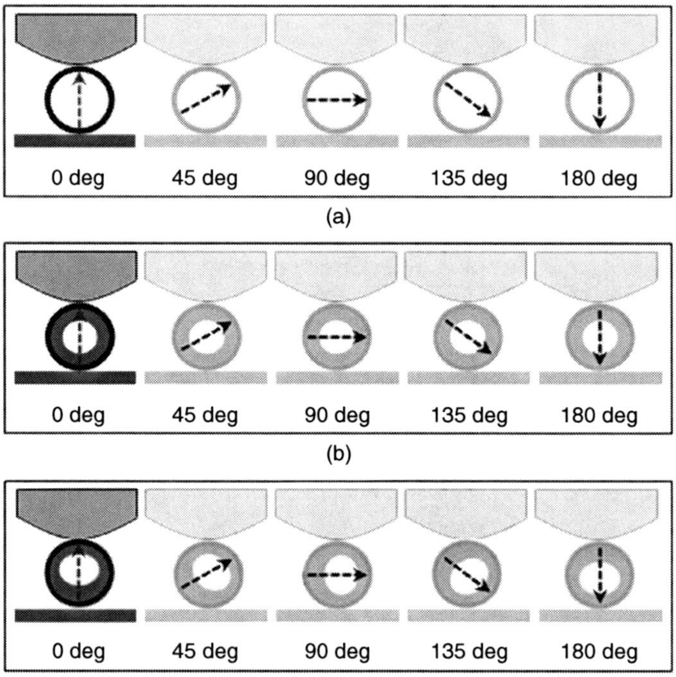

FIGURE 9.53 Schematic representation of models considered to investigate the effect of rolling. (*a*) healthy artery, (*b*) axisymmetric stenotic artery, and (*c*) non-axisymmetric stenotic artery.
Abouei et al., "A Novel Method in Exploration of Arteries Inside a Tissue and Assessment of the Arteries by Computational Approach," Proceedings of the IEEE/ASME International Conference on Advanced Intelligent Mechatronics (AIM), Montreal, Canada, July 2010, © IEEE.

side of each model at every 45 degrees of rotation. The following results were elicited from the stress graphs shown in Figs. 9.54, 9.55, and 9.56.

As shown in Fig. 9.54, there is not only an increase (overshoot) in the stress graphs that are taken from models *a* and *b* but, also, the number of changes in stress peaks versus time. Hence, it can be concluded that models *a* and *b* consist of an artery. Although the peaks in model *b* appear to be the same at different times, if we zoom into part of the graph, it can be seen that they are not the same. The difference between the maximum and minimum stress at this location was recorded to be 22.6 Pa.

Also, as shown in Fig. 9.55, in the stress graphs taken from the bottom surface of the finger in models *a* and *b*, the peak point in each stress graph, and their dependence on time, could be observed. Furthermore, comparing the two graphs, it was seen that the amplitude of the stress peaks of models *a* and *b* is different at the same times. This is because the stiffness of the stenotic artery is larger than that of a healthy artery and this is one of the useful criteria for surgeons in diagnosing arterial stenosis during surgery. Also, it can be observed from Fig. 9.55 that the amplitude of stress variation versus time in model *a* is larger than model *b*. This is due to the fact that the stenotic artery has a larger and stiffer wall than the healthy artery which reduces the transmitting effect of

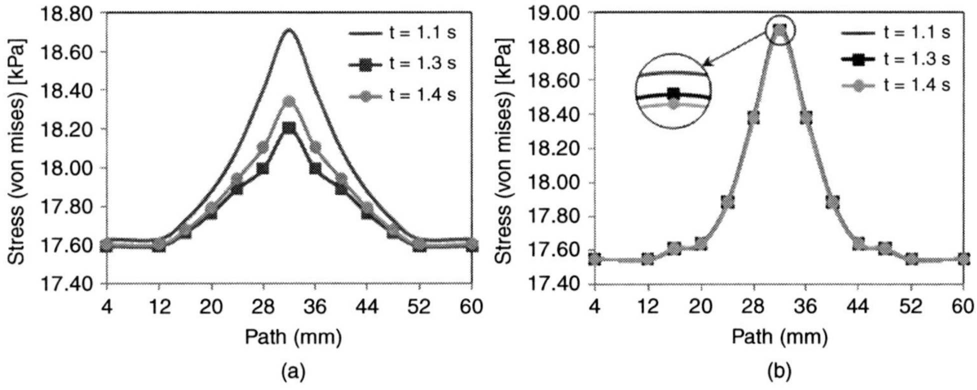

FIGURE 9.54 The stress graphs of the top surface of the soft tissue models including (*a*) healthy, and (*b*) stenotic artery. [From Abouei (2010),[48] used by permission.]

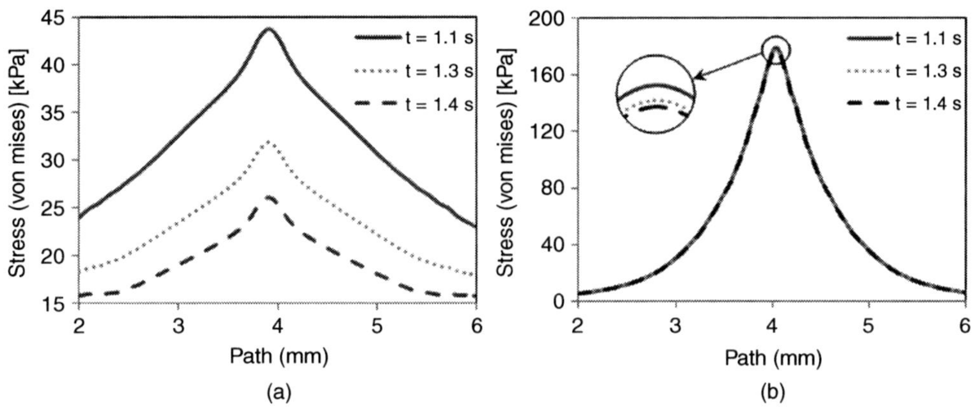

FIGURE 9.55 The stress graphs of the bottom surface of the finger in models of single (*a*) healthy, and (*b*) stenotic artery. [From Abouei (2010),[48] used by permission.]

blood pressure from the inner surface of artery wall to its outer surface. So, it can be concluded, that the separation of a healthy artery from a stenotic artery is possible by comparing their stiffness and pulse intensity.[52]

Moreover, when simulating the rolling process of arteries by the surgeon for better diagnosis of arterial disease during surgery, as shown in Fig. 9.53, the results presented in Fig. 9.56 showed that the amount of stress the surgeon feels on the bottom surface of her/his finger does not change in every step of the rolling process for a healthy or axisymmetric stenotic artery. It should be noted that this value for a stenotic artery is larger than that of a healthy one. However, in an artery with non-axisymmetric stenosis, the surgeon does not sense the same value of stress when rolling the artery.

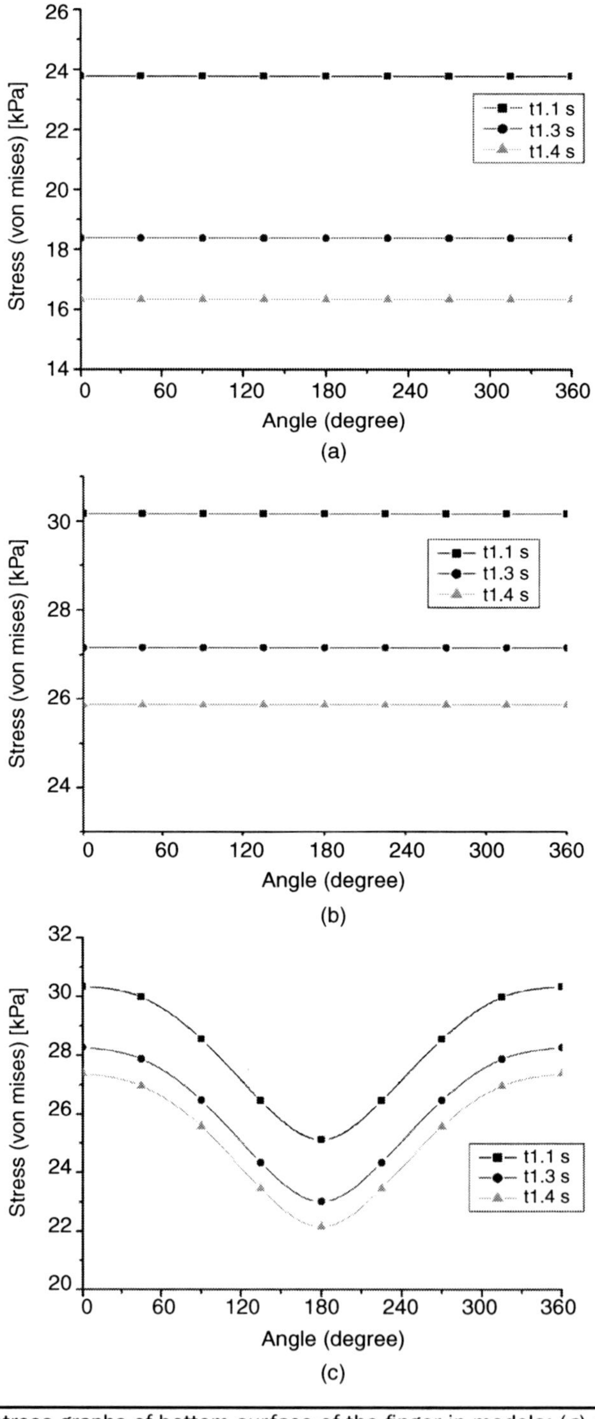

Figure 9.56 The stress graphs of bottom surface of the finger in models: (*a*) a healthy artery, (*b*) a axisymmetric stenotic artery, and (*c*) a non-axisymmetric stenotic artery.

Abouei et al., "A Novel Method in Exploration of Arteries Inside a Tissue and Assessment of the Arteries by Computational Approach," Proceedings of the IEEE/ASME International Conference on Advanced Intelligent Mechatronics (AIM), Montreal, Canada, July 2010, © IEEE.

Parameter	Value	Parameter	Value
Elastic modulus of soft tissue	100 kPa	Inside diameter of the artery	4 mm
Elastic modulus of artery	400 kPa	Depth of the artery	10 mm
Finger indentation	4 mm	Artery thickness	0.56 mm

From Abouei (2010),[48] used by permission.

Table 9.11 Values of Different Parameters of the Basic Model

Investigation of the Effect of Changing Different Parameters on Detection of an Artery To determine whether or not the proposed system is able to detect an artery in different situations, the effects of the parameters of a model consisting of a healthy artery are investigated. These parameters include the artery diameter, its elastic modulus, the artery depth, and the tissue indentation caused by the finger displacement on artery detection. Table 9.11 shows the different parameters considered for the basic model.

Figures 9.57 to 9.60 display the tactile map showing the difference between the maximum and minimum stresses which has been considered as being the intensity of the arterial pulse. Analyzing the graphs, it can be concluded that:

- Increasing the artery depth in the tissue causes the pulse intensity to become smaller and finally to disappear. This means that, in practice, the farther the artery is from the tissue surface, the more difficult it becomes for the surgeon to feel the arterial pulse. Hence, artificial tactile sensing could be considered as being a more appropriate approach in the detection of superficial arteries.
- Increasing the indentation causes the difference between the maximum and minimum stresses to become more noticeable. It should be considered that the finger displacement in modeling was less than the amount by which the artery would collapse.

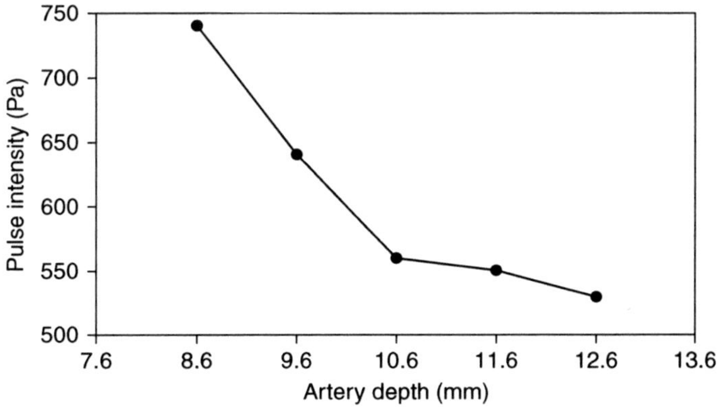

Figure 9.57 Effect of changing the depth of the artery on pulse intensity detected on the surface of the tissue. [From Abouei (2010),[48] used by permission.]

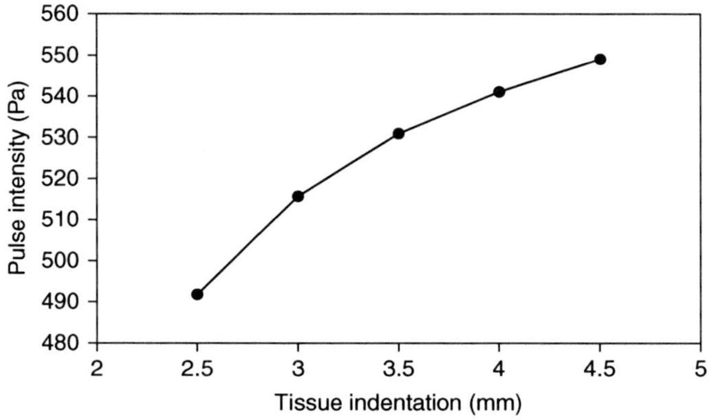

Figure 9.58 Effect of changing the indentation of the finger on pulse intensity detected on the surface of the tissue. [From Abouei (2010),[48] used by permission.]

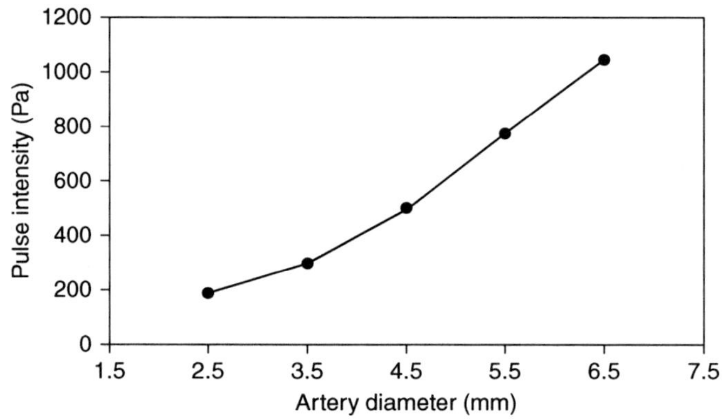

Figure 9.59 Effect of changing the diameter of the artery on pulse intensity detected on the surface of the tissue. [From Abouei (2010),[48] used by permission.]

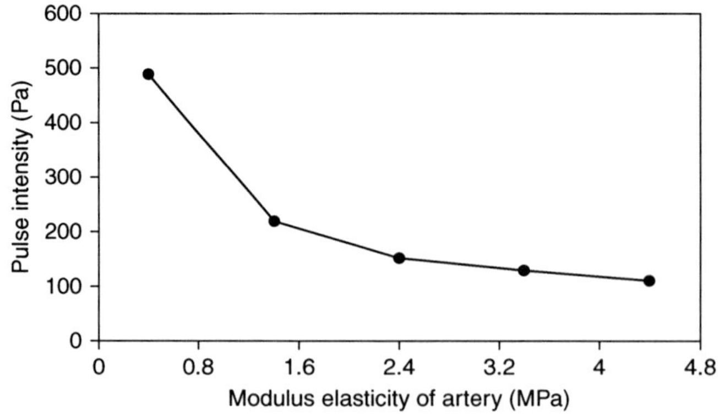

Figure 9.60 Effect of changing the modulus of elasticity of the artery on pulse intensity detected on the surface of the tissue. [From Abouei (2010),[48] used by permission.]

- It is evidently a lot faster and easier to find an artery with larger diameters.
- Increasing the elastic modulus of the artery reduces the pulse intensity. It is a lot easier to find an artery in the breast tissue than in a muscular tissue.

Sensor Structure Capable of Artery Detecting Some experimental setups have been used to determine the existence of an artery in soft tissue. In 1994, Peine et al. designed a system that was able to locate hidden and inaccessible arteries.[53] As shown in Fig. 9.61, the system consisted of an array of sensors that were installed at the tip of a long probe 10 mm in diameter. During surgery, the surgeon pushed the probe to the surface of the tissue and, by analyzing and processing the stress distribution on the surface of the probe at each step, the system detected a pulsatile flow wave. The results were then shown in such a way that the surgeon could utilize the information for the purposes of decision making. In this sensor, when contacting the tissue, the sensor surface pushes the silicon rubber which, in turn, decreases the distance between copper strips thereby producing a signal that is used by other parts of the system, of which a block diagram is shown in Fig. 9.62.

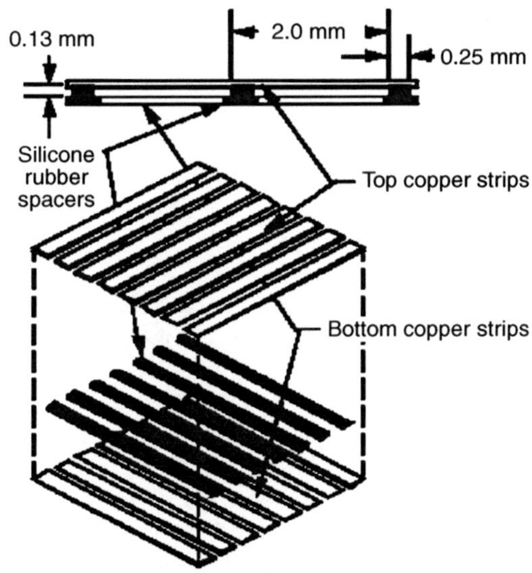

FIGURE 9.61 A front and exploded view of the tactile array sensor.

Peine et al. "A Palpation System for Artery Localization in Laparoscopic Surgery," 1st International Symposium on Medical Robotics and Computer Assisted Surgery, Pittsburgh, September 1994. Used by permission.

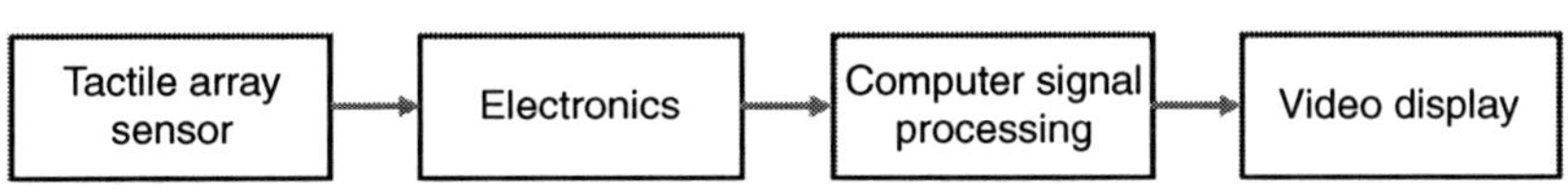

FIGURE 9.62 A block diagram of the system.

Peine et al. "A Palpation System for Artery Localization in Laparoscopic Surgery," 1st International Symposium on Medical Robotics and Computer Assisted Surgery, Pittsburgh, September 1994. Used by permission.

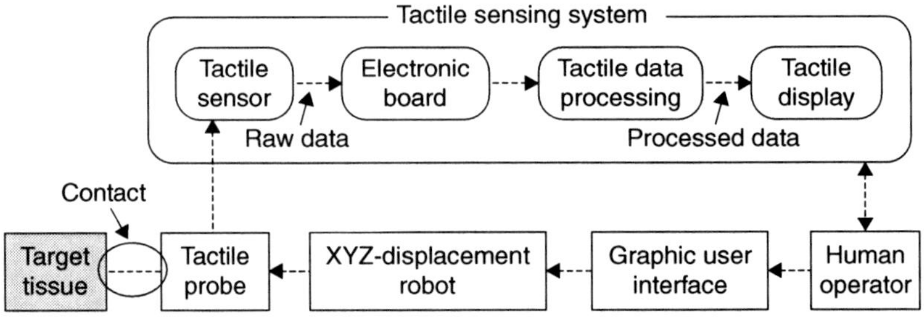

FIGURE 9.63 The components of the tactile sensing system.
"Modeling, Constructing, and Testing of a Novel Tactile System to Detect Arterial Stenosis by Imitating Surgeon's Palpation," Abouei et al., *International Journal of Academic Research*, vol. 2, no. 6, pp. 120–125, 2010. Used by permission.

In 2002, Beasley et al. designed a copper capacitance-type sensor that, by palpating the surface of the tissue, could detect the path of an inside artery.[54] The tactile sensor is placed on the tissue by a surgical robot. Changing the distance between two copper sheets produces a signal that can detect the existence of an artery. Then, some predefined algorithms predict potential paths of the artery but if, after moving to a predicted place, the artery is no longer detected, a reverse mechanism returns the sensor to its previous location.

Recently, a tactile sensor was designed by Abouei et al. that can detect stenosis in arteries and is able to distinguish between a healthy artery and a stenotic artery. This system is explained in following section.

A Novel Tactile System to Detect Arterial Stenosis by Limiting Surgeon's Palpation The main components of the proposed Tactile Arterial Stenosis Detector,[49] are shown in Fig. 9.63. The main part of the tactile probe consists of a 350-g strain gauge load cell with an accuracy of ±0.5 g. The experimental setup, together with component details, is shown in Fig. 9.64.

The tactile display system was designed using MATLAB software. Data was transmitted between the electronic board and the computer via a serial port. Additionally, four similar silicone tubes were prepared in order to simulate four different arteries including a healthy and a 30 percent stenotic artery extracted from adjacent tissue (models 1 and 2, respectively) and a healthy and 30 percent stenotic artery extracted from inside the tissue (models 3 and 4, respectively). To simulate the mechanical characteristics of the soft tissue, paraffin gel was used. To imitate the pulsatile effect of blood pressure inside the tubes, a peristaltic pump was used to push the water for a period of 1 second. Then, the robot scanned each tube using a tactile probe.

Experimental Results In the force graphs taken from models 1 and 2 at time intervals of 1.35 seconds (maximum water pressure) and 1.55 seconds (minimum water pressure), we observe that the graphs of these two models, as shown in Figs. 9.65*a* and *b*, are time dependent and the force graph of model 2 has a peak. The reason for this overshoot is the existence of stenosis in the tube of model 2. The values of the pulse intensity for models 1 and 2 near the 30 mm point were 7 grams and 2 grams, respectively. Also, in models 3 and 4, two time-dependent force graphs were observed as

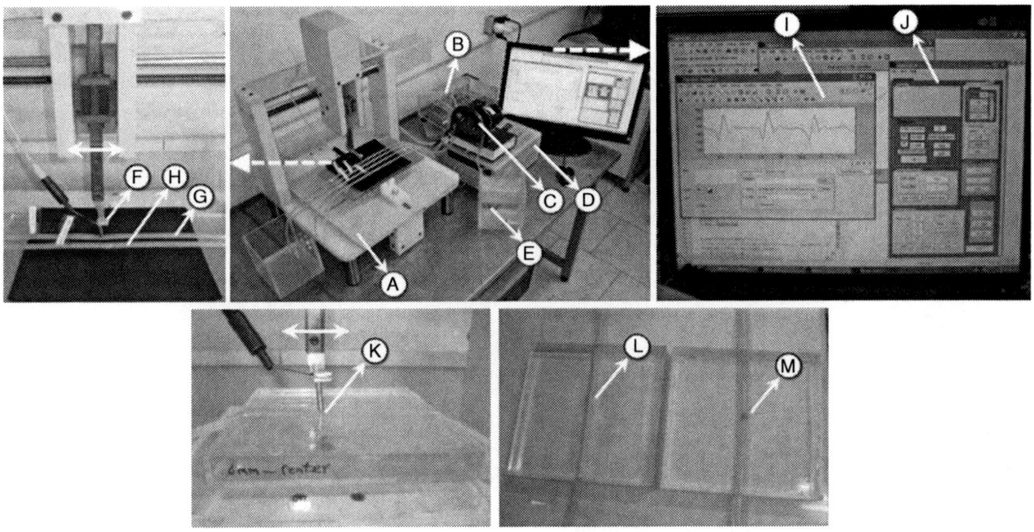

Figure 9.64 Photographs of the experimental setup: A. XYZ-displacement robot, B. Electronic board, C. Peristaltic pump, D. Power supply, E. Water tank, F. Strain gauge load cell, G. The silicone tube as a healthy artery, H. The silicone tube with 30 percent narrowing as a 30 percent stenotic artery, I. Tactile display, J. Graphic user interface, K. The contact of tactile probe and paraffin gel including a silicone tube, L. A frame of paraffin gel including a silicone tube, and M. A frame of paraffin gel including a silicone tube with 30 percent narrowing

"Modeling, Constructing, and Testing of a Novel Tactile System to Detect Arterial Stenosis by Imitating Surgeon's Palpation," Abouei et al., *International Journal of Academic Research*, vol. 2, no. 6, pp. 120–125, 2010. Used by permission.

shown in Figs. 9.65*c* and *d*. Also, it was found that the maximum force for a stenotic tube is larger than a tube without any narrowing because the stiffness of the stenotic tube is larger. The greater the maximum force, the more the percentage of stenosis. Moreover, it was perceived from these graphs that the pulse intensity of model 3 is larger than model 4 due to the fact that the stenotic tube had a thicker wall than the other tube, thereby reducing the transmitting effect of the water pressure from the inner surface of the tube wall to its outer surface.

9.8 An Instrument for Esophagectomy

Esophageal cancer, which is one of the most common cancers worldwide, causes adhesion of the esophagus to the surrounding tissues including the aorta and the lungs. There are several approaches to treat esophageal cancer. The surgeon first usually tries to cure the disease by chemotherapy and/or radiation therapy. However, if the cancer has developed widely, surgery is necessary to remove the esophagus. The two most common surgical procedures to treat esophageal cancer are transthoracic esophagectomy and transhiatal esophagectomy. Transthoracic esophagectomy is the older approach which involves an abdominal incision and a thoracotomy. During this type of surgery, it is necessary to make a wide incision in the abdominal part of the skin so that the surgeon can access the esophagus

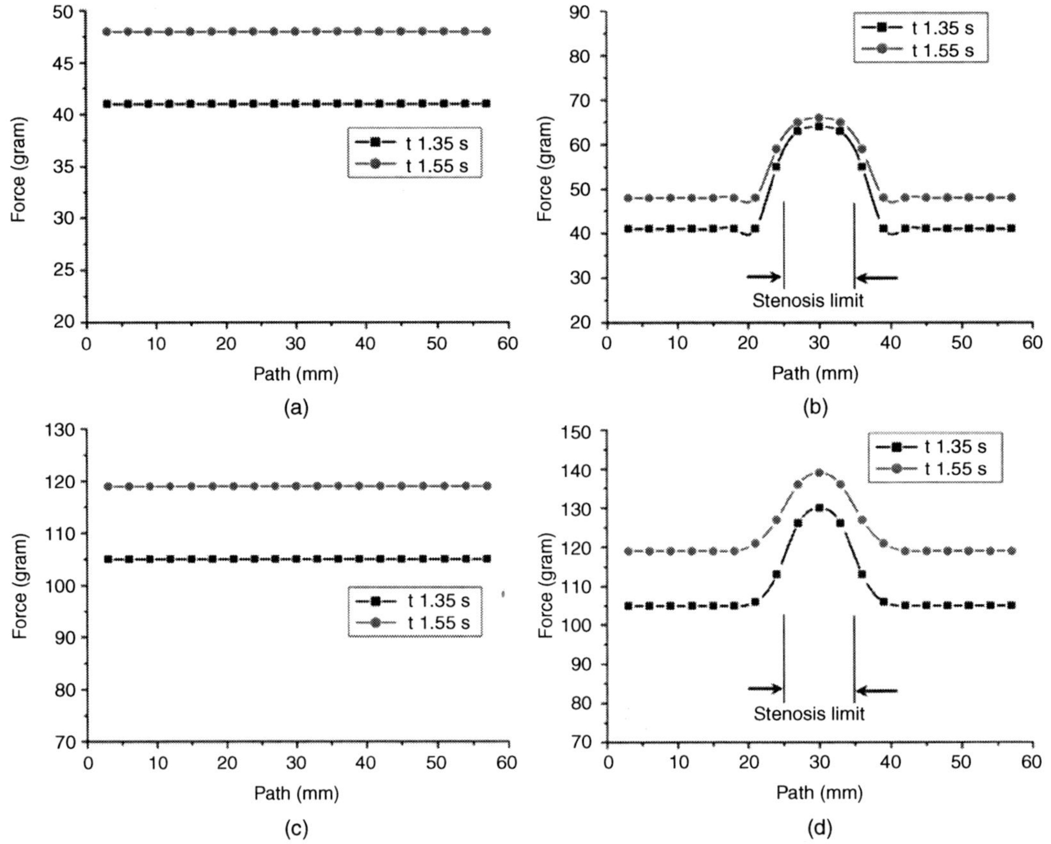

FIGURE 9.65 The force graph of load cell for (*a*) model 1, (*b*) model 2, (*c*) model 3, and (*d*) model 4. Modeling, Constructing, and Testing of a Novel Tactile System to Detect Arterial Stenosis by Imitating Surgeon's Palpation, Abouei et al., *International Journal of Academic Research*, vol. 2, no. 6, pp. 120–125, 2010. Used by permission.

and proceed to dissect it from the surrounding tissues. The drastic nature of this operation causes a great deal of trauma to the patient including blood loss and prolonged recovery time and can even, in a few cases, lead to post-operative mortality. To avoid these drawbacks, in the 1970s a new method was introduced by Orringer who named the procedure transhiatal esophagectomy.[55] In this procedure, most of the lower esophagus and uppermost portion of the stomach are dissected and the remaining parts sutured together to preserve digestive tract functioning. Transhiatal esophagectomy involves both an abdominal incision and a cervical incision. During the operation, the surgeon opens the diaphragmatic hiatus and mobilizes the esophagus by careful manual dissection up into the thoracic cavity.[56]

Since this technique avoids the necessity of making a large abdominal incision, it can reduce post-operative morbidities and make the recovery faster. However, during transhiatal esophagectomy, the surgeon needs to enter his/her hand into the patient's thorax and, considering the large size of the surgeon's hand compared to the finite volume of the thorax, there is always an enormous risk of damage to the delicate biological structures within the thorax, such as the aorta artery, lungs, airways, and trachea.[57]

To minimize this risk, Farkoush and Najarian proposed a robotic hand only one quarter the size of the surgeon's but which could, nonetheless, function just as equally during transhiatal esophagectomy.[57] The proposed device, that has fingers consisting of rotational joints and which can sheer and dissect tissue, is inserted into the thorax from the distal part of esophagus through a 5-cm large incision in the abdomen. It then surrounds the esophagus and goes up to its proximal part to perform the dissection process. The instrument is equipped with a lever that is controlled by the surgeon who ensures accurate control on the movement of the instrument's dynamic fingers. An isometric view of the proposed instrument is shown in Fig. 9.66.

The instrument head consists of two hollow semi-cylinders, each of which has five dynamic fingers of which each has a rotational joint and a synchronized radial motion as shown in Fig. 9.67. These two parts are first unhooked and are able to attach and turn into a hollow cylinder that surrounds the esophagus whenever the surgeon activates the locking mechanism. In this way, at the beginning, the surgical instrument surrounds the esophagus radially and prepares to dissect the adhesive tissues.

In the next step, when the instrument is situated in the distal part of the esophagus, an axle-arm mechanism changes the lever movement to a linear displacement which, in turn, changes the dynamic diameter of the fingers from 15 to 70 mm. This provides the ability to perform environmental dissection of the adhesive tissues while going ahead. In order to transfer the lever motion to fingers, a cable drive mechanism is used. Figure 9.68 shows how the proposed instrument dissects the adhesive tissues. Sheering the tissue up to about 7 cm and increasing the outside diameter of the fingers gives the instrument the ability to dissect the adhesions between the esophagus and the sticky area around it.

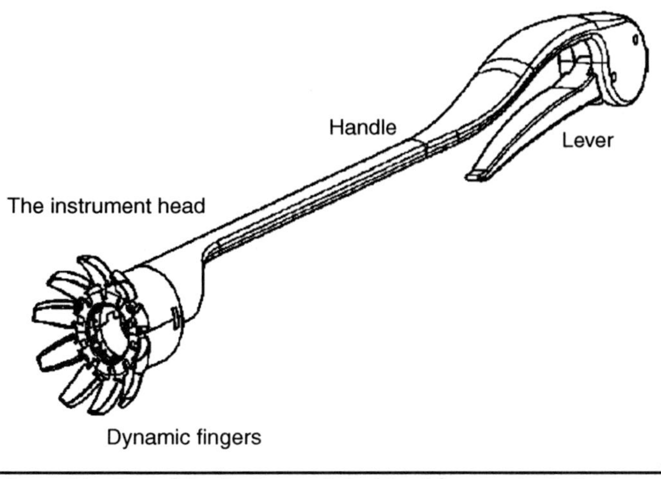

FIGURE 9.66 An isometric view of the instrument designed for esophagectomy.

Reprinted from Medical Hypotheses, vol. 73, Hajizadeh Farkoush and Najarian. "Can Surgeon's Hand be Replaced with a Smart Surgical Instrument in Esophagectomy," pp. 735–740, Copyright © 2009, with permission from Elsevier.

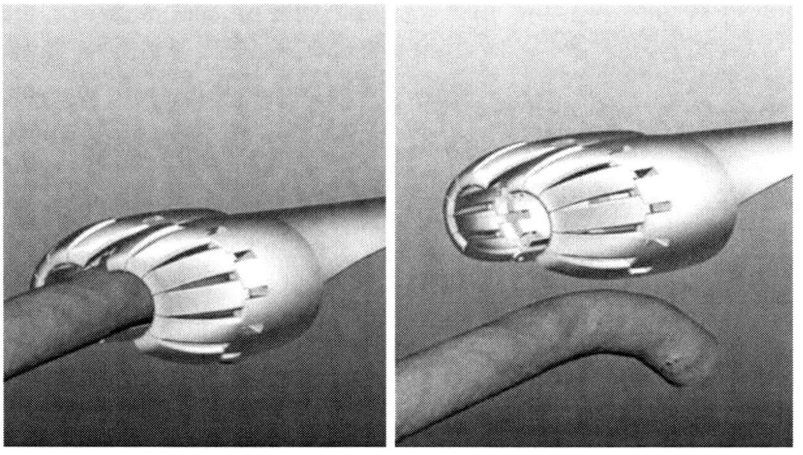

FIGURE 9.67 Two semi-cylindrical-shaped parts of the head of the instrument; these two parts are unhooked, after that they are placed around the esophagus, a locking mechanism changes them to a hollow cylinder.

Reprinted from Medical Hypotheses, vol. 73, Hajizadeh Farkoush and Najarian. "Can Surgeon's Hand be Replaced with a Smart Surgical Instrument in Esophagectomy," pp. 735–740, Copyright © 2009, with permission from Elsevier.

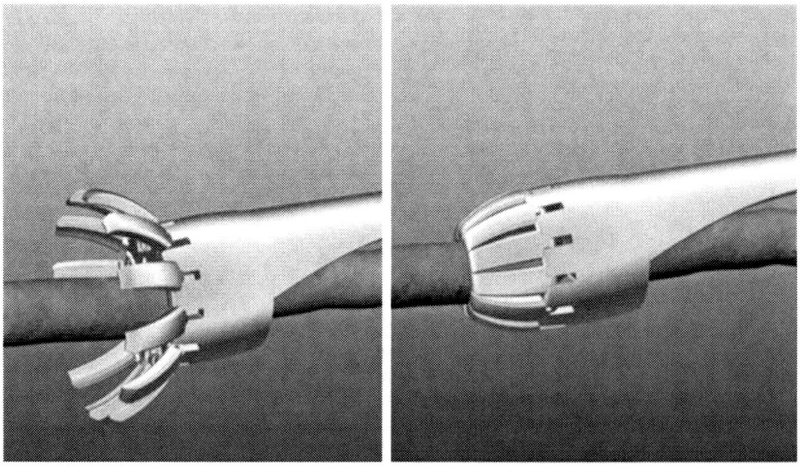

FIGURE 9.68 Dissecting process of surrounding tissues from esophagus.

Reprinted from Medical Hypotheses, vol. 73, Hajizadeh Farkoush and Najarian. "Can Surgeon's Hand Be Replaced with a Smart Surgical Instrument in Esophagectomy," pp. 735–740, Copyright © 2009, with permission from Elsevier.

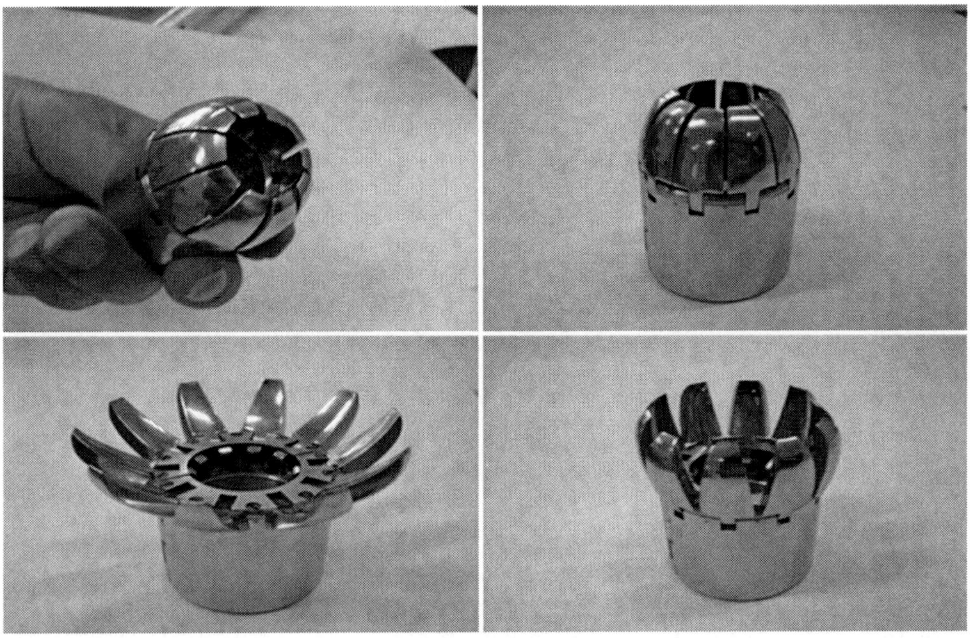

Figure 9.69 The fabricated prototype of the proposed instrument in different positions. Reprinted from Medical Hypotheses, vol. 73, Hajizadeh Farkoush and Najarian. "Can Surgeon's Hand Be Replaced with a Smart Surgical Instrument in Esophagectomy," pp. 735–740, Copyright © 2009, with permission from Elsevier.

Figure 9.69 shows the fabricated prototype of the proposed instrument in different positions. The prototype was made of medical grade stainless steel.

References

1. F. Focacci, M. Piccigallo, O. Tonet, G. Megali, A. Pietrabissa, and P. Dario. "Lightweight Handheld Robot for Laparoscopic Surgery," *IEEE International Conference on Robotics and Automation*, 2007, pp. 599–604.
2. S. Mosafer Khoorjestan. "Design and Construction of a Snake-like Robotic Instrument for Minimally Invasive Surgery," M.Sc. Thesis, 2009, Amirkabir University of Technology, Iran.
3. S. Mosafer Khoorjestan, S. Najarian, N. Simforoosh, and S. Hajizadeh Farkoush. "Design and Modeling of a Novel Flexible Surgical Instrument Applicable in Minimally Invasive Surgery," *International Journal of Natural and Engineering Sciences*, vol. 4, no. 1, 2010, pp. 49–56.
4. http://www.NKUIC.com/ Kidney & Urologic Diseases A-Z List of Topics and Titles: "Kidney Stones in Adults."
5. S. Holmes and H. N. Whitfield. "The Current Status of Lithotripsy," *Journal of Urology*, vol. 68, 1991, pp. 337–344.
6. E. Afshari, S. Najarian, N. Simforoosh, and S. Hajizadeh Farkoush. "Design and Fabrication of a Novel Tactile Sensory System Applicable in Artificial Palpation," *Minimally Invasive Therapy and Allied Technologies*, vol. 20, no. 1, 2011, pp. 22–29.
7. A. El-Baz, R. Fahmi, S. Yuksel, A. A. Farag, W. Miller, M. A. El-Ghar, and T. Eldiasty. "A New CAD System for the Evaluation of Kidney Diseases Using DCE-MRI," *Medical Image Computing and Computer-Assisted Intervention Journal*, 2006, pp. 446–453.

8. N. P. Cohen and H. N. Whitfield. "Mechanical Testing of Urinary Calculi," *World Journal of Urology*, vol. 11, 1993, pp. 13–18.
9. E. Afshari, S. Najarian, N. Simforoosh, and S. Hajizadeh Farkoush. "Evaluation of a New Method for Detection of Kidney Stone during Laparoscopy Using 3D Conceptual Modeling," *International Journal of Biological and Life Sciences*, vol. 8, no. 1, 2012, pp. 56–61.
10. E. Afshari, S. Najarian, and N. Simforoosh. "Application of Artificial Tactile Sensing Approach in Kidney-Stone-Removal Laparoscopy," *Bio-Medical Materials and Engineering*, vol. 20, 2010, pp. 261–267.
11. http://www.cancer.org/downloads/STT/2008CAFFfinalsecured.pdf. "Cancer Facts & Figures," *American Cancer Society*, 2008.
12. J. Zeng, Y. Wang, M. T. Freedman, and S. K. Mum. "Finger Tracking for Breast Palpation Quantification Using Color Image Features," *SPIE J. of Opt. Eng.*, vol. 36, 1997, pp. 3455–3461.
13. A. J. Evans, A. R. M. Wilson, H. C. Burrell, I. O. Ellis, and S. E. Pinder. "Mammographic Features of Ducta l Sarcinoma in Situ (DCIS) Present on Previous Mammography," *Clinical Radiology*, vol. 54, 1999, pp. 644–646.
14. B. J. Kane, M. R. Cutkosky, and G. T. Kavacs. "Compatible Traction Stress Sensor for Use in High-Resolution Tactile Imaging," *Sensors and Actuators A-Physical*, vol. 54, 1996, pp. 511–516.
15. S. Najarian, J. Dargahi, and V. Mirjalili. "Detecting Embedded Objects Using Haptics with Applications in Artificial Palpation of Masses," *Sensors & Materials*, vol. 18, 2006, pp. 215–229.
16. S. Najarian, J. Dargahi, and A. Abouei Mehrizi. *Artificial Tactile Sensing in Biomedical Engineering*, McGraw-Hill, USA, 2009.
17. A. Mojra, S. Najarian, S. M. Towliat Kashani, F. Panahi, and M. Yaghmaei. "A Novel Haptic Robotic Viscogram for Characterizing Viscoelastic Behavior of Breast Tissue in Clinical Examinations," *International Journal of Medical Robotics and Computer Assisted Surgery*, 2011, In Press.
18. A. Mojra. "Design and Construction of an Intelligent Tactile System with Application in Clinical Breast Examinations," Ph.D. Thesis, 2011, Amirkabir University of Technology, Iran.
19. A. Mojra, S. Najarian, S. M. Hosseini, S. M. Towliat Kashani, and F. Panahi. "Abnormal Mass Detection in a Real Breast Model: A Computational Tactile Sensing Approach," *Proceedings of the 11th World Congress on Medical Physics and Biomedical Engineering (IFMBE)*, Munich, Germany, 2009.
20. I. Jatoi, M. Kaufmann, and J. Y. Petit. *Atlas of Breast Surgery*, Berlin Heidelberg: Springer-Verlag, 2006.
21. A. Mojra, S. Najarian, S. M. Towliat Kashani, F. Panahi, and M. A. Tehrani. "A Novel Robotic Tactile Mass Detector with Application in Clinical Breast Examination," *Minimally Invasive Therapy and Allied Technologies*, 2011, In Press.
22. P. S. Wellman and R. D. Howe. "Mechanical Properties of Breast Tissue in Compression," Harvard BioRobotics Laboratory Technical Report #99003, 1999.
23. F. C. Brunicardi. *Schwartz's Principles of Surgery*, 8th ed., McGraw-Hill, USA, 2005.
24. N. Nasseri, F. Almasganj, S. Najarian, and S. H. Farkoush. "A Novel Experimental Analysis for the Scientific Study and Evaluation of Sprained Ankle," *Journal of Medical Technology and Physical Therapy*, vol. 23, no. 1, 2011.
25. C. Bauckhage, J. K. Tsotsos, and F. E. Bunn. "Automatic Detection of Abnormal Gait," *Image and Vision Computing Journal*, vol. 27, 2009, pp. 108–115.
26. M. S. Muniz and J. Nadal. "Application of Principal Component Analysis in Vertical Ground Reaction Force to Discriminate Normal and Abnormal Gait," *Gait. Posture*, vol. 29, 2009, pp. 31–35.
27. L. M. Schutte, U. Narayanan, J. L. Stout, P. Selber, J. R. Gage, and M. H. Schwartz. "An Index for Quantifying Deviations from Normal Gait," *Gait. Posture*, vol. 11, 2000, pp. 25–31.
28. N. Nasseri. "Design and Construction of a Novel Sensor Element for Dynamic Foot-Pressure Signal Processing," M.Sc. Thesis, 2009, Amirkabir University of Technology, Iran.
29. N. Nasseri, F. Almasganj, S. Najarian, and S. H. Farkoush. "An Embedded Insole, Applicable in Signal Processing: Sprained Ankle Assessment," *International Journal of Intelligent Information Technology Application*, vol. 2, no. 4, 2009, pp. 144–150.
30. A. J. Worth and R. C. Spencer. "A Neural Network for Tactile Sensing: The Hertzian Contact Problem," *IEEE Transactions on Systems, Man, and Cybernetics*, vol. 22, 1992, pp. 177–182.
31. D. T. Fong, Y. Y. Chan, Y. Hong, P. S. Yung, K. Y. Fung, and K. M. Chan. "A Three-Pressure-Sensor (3PS) System for Monitoring Ankle Supination Torque during Sport Motions," *Journal of Biomechanics*, vol. 41, 2008, pp. 2562–2566.

32. K. R. Kaufman, J. A. Levine, R. H. Brey, S. K. McCrady, D. J. Padgett, and M. J. Joyner. "Energy Expenditure and Activity of Transfemoral Amputees Using Mechanical and Microprocessor-Controlled Prosthetic Knees," *Archives of Physical Medicine and Rehabilitation*, vol. 89, 2008, pp. 1380–1385.
33. G. H. Traugh, P. J. Corcoran, and R. L. Reyes. "Energy Expenditure of Ambulation in Patients with Transfemoral Amputation," *Archives of Physical Medicine and Rehabilitation*, vol. 56, 1975, pp. 67–71.
34. D. A. Winter. *Biomechanics of Motor Control and Human Gait: Normal, Elderly and Pathological*, 2nd ed.University of Waterloo Press, 1991.
35. R. Waters, J. Perry, D. Antonelli, and H. Hislop. "Energy Cost of Walking Amputees: the Influence of Level of Amputation," *Journal of Bone and Joint Surgery*, vol. 58, 1976, pp. 42–46.
36. Y. Dabiri, S. Najarian, M. R. Eslami, S. Zahedi, H. Farahpour, and R. Moradi Haghighat. "Comparison of Passive and Active Prosthetic Knee Joint Kinematics during Swing Phase of Gait," *Proceedings of 17th Iranian Conference on Biomedical Engineering*, Isfahan, Iran, 2010.
37. J. Perry. *Gait Analysis*, SLACK, Thorofare, NJ, 1992.
38. Y. Dabiri, S. Najarian, S. Zahedi, D. Moser, and E. Shirzad. "Muscle Contributions in the Swing Phase of Transfemoral Amputee Gait: An Inverse Dynamics Approach," *Research Journal of Biological Sciences*, vol. 4, 2009, pp. 1076–1084.
39. S. J. Piazza and S. L. Delp. "The Influence of Muscles on Knee Flexion during the Swing Phase of Gait," *Journal of Biomechanics*, vol. 29, 1992, pp. 723–733.
40. F. Sup, A. Bohara, and M. Goldfarb. "Design and Control of a Powered Transfemoral Prosthesis," *The International Journal of Robotics Research*, vol. 27, 2008, pp. 263–273.
41. F. C. Anderson and M. G. Pandy. "Static and dynamic optimization solutions for gait are practically equivalent," *Journal of biomechanics*, vol. 34, 2001, pp. 153–161.
42. S. L. Delp. "Surgery Simulation: A Computer Graphics System to Analyze and Design Musculoskeletal Reconstructions of the Lower Limb," Ph.D. Thesis, 1990, Stanford University, CA, USA.
43. Y. Dabiri. "Design, Construction and Analysis of an Active Prosthetic Knee Joint Powered by the Artificial Muscle," Ph.D. Thesis, 2010, Amirkabir University of Technology, Iran.
44. D. G. Smith, J. M. Michael, and J. H. Bowker, (Eds.). *Atlas of Amputations and Limb Deficiencies: Surgical, Prosthetic, and Rehabilitation Principles*, 3d ed., American Academy of Orthopaedic Surgeons, 2004.
45. A. Abouei Mehrizi, S. Najarian, M. Moini, and F. Tabatabai Ghomshe. "Modeling of Tactile Detection of an Artery in a Soft Tissue by Finite Element Method," *American Journal of Applied Sciences*, vol. 5, no. 2, 2008, pp. 83–88.
46. J. Dargahi and S. Najarian. "Advances in Tactile Sensors Design, Manufacturing, and Its Impact on Robotics Applications–a Review," *Industrial Robot: An Introduction Journal*, vol. 32/3, 2005, pp. 268–281.
47. J. Dargahi and S. Najarian. "Human Tactile Perception as a Standard for Artificial Tactile Sensing-a review," *International Journal of Medical Robotics and Computer Assisted Surgery*, vol. 1, 2004, pp. 23–35.
48. A. Abouei Mehrizi. "Modeling, Constructing and Testing of a Tactile Sensing System for Detecting Arteries and Diagnosis of Stenosis in a Peripheral Tissue," Ph.D. Thesis, 2010, Amirkabir University of Technology, Iran.
49. A. Abouei, S. Najarian, and M. Moini. "Modeling, Constructing, and Testing of a Novel Tactile System to Detect Arterial Stenosis by Imitating Surgeon's Palpation," *International Journal of Academic Research*, vol. 2, no. 6, 2010, pp. 120–125.
50. A. Ansari Benam. "Experimental Study of Blood Flow and FSI Analysis of Stenotic Arteries," M.Sc. Thesis, 2007, Amirkabir University of Technology, Iran.
51. A. Abouei Mehrizi, S. Najarian, M. Moini, J. Dargahi, and R. Ahmadi. "A Novel Method in Exploration of Arteries Inside a Tissue and Assessment of the Arteries by Computational Approach," *Proceedings of the IEEE/ASME International Conference on Advanced Intelligent Mechatronics*, 2010, Montreal, Canada.
52. A. Abouei Mehrizi, S. Najarian, R. Khodambashi, and S. Dehkhoda. "A Novel Method of Tactile Assessment of Arteries Using Computational Approach," *International Journal of Academic Research*, In Press.
53. W. J. Peine, J. S. Son, and R. D. Howe. "A Palpation System for Artery Localization in Laparoscopic Surgery," *1st International Symposium in Medical Robotics and Computer Assisted Surgery*, 1994, pp. 22–24.

54. R. A. Beasley and R. D. Howe. "Tactile Tracking of Arteries in Robotic Surgery," *proceedings of the 2002 IEEE International Conference on Robotics & Automation*, 2002, Washington DC.
55. M. B. Orringer. "Transhiatal Esophagectomy without Thoracotomy for Carcinoma of the Thoracic Esophagus," *Annals of Surgery*, vol. 200, 1984, pp. 282–288.
56. D. J. Mackenzie, P. K. Pepperell, and K. G. Billingsley. "Care of Patients after Esophagectomy," *Critical Care Nursing*, vol. 24, 2004, pp. 16–31.
57. S. Hajizadeh Farkoush, and S. Najarian. "Can Surgeon's Hand Be Replaced with a Smart Surgical Instrument in Esophagectomy?" *Medical Hypothesis*, vol. 73, 2009, pp. 735–740.

Abbreviations and Symbols

Abbreviations

A/D	analog-to-digital
AC	alternating current
Acc	accuracy
ADC	analog-to-digital converter
AI	artificial intelligence
ALU	arithmetic logic unit
ANFIS	adaptive network-based fuzzy inference system
ANN	artificial neural networks
AvS_i	average stiffness
CBE	clinical breast examination
ChemFET	chemical field-effect transistor
CPR	cycles per revolution
CPU	central processing unit
CT	computed tomography
D/A	digital-to-analog
D/D	digital-to-digital
DAC	digital-to-analog converter
DC	direct current
DQE	detector quantum efficiency
DSP	digital signal processor
EEG	electroencephalogram
ENFET	enzyme field-effect transistor
EPROM	erasable programmable read only memory
FALCON	fuzzy adaptive learning control network
FDA	food and drug administration

FL	focused laser
FMRI	functional magnetic resonance imaging
FS	input full scale
FSO	full-scale output
FSR	force sensing resistor
I/O	input to output
I^2C	inter-integrated circuit
IC	integrated circuit
ICU	intensive care unit
IPMC	ionic polymer-metal composite
ISFET	ion-sensitive field-effect transistor
JSPMI	Japanese society for the promotion of machine industry
LED	light-emitting diode
LVDT	linear variable differential transformer
MBL	minigram beam load cell
MEMS	micro-electro-mechanical systems
MIS	minimally invasive surgery
MLP	multilayer perceptron
MR	magnetoresistance
MRI	magnetic resonance imaging
MTBF	mean time between failures
NEFCON	neuro-fuzzy control
NNS	neural network-based screening
$normS_i$	normalized stiffness
NPV	negative predictive value
NTC	negative temperature coefficient
PC	personal computer
PID	proportional-integral-derivative
PPV	positive predictive value
pred	predecessor (parent)
PS	pressure sensor
PTC	positive temperature coefficient
PVDF or PVF_2	polyvinylidene fluoride
PWM	pulse width modulation
RAM	random access memory
RF	radio frequency

RGB	red, green, and blue
Robo-Tac-BMI	robotic tactile breast mass identifier
ROM	read-only memory
rpm	revolutions per minute
RTD	resistance temperature detector
RVDT	rotary variable differential transformer
SBE	self-breast examination
SCARA	selective compliant articulated robot arm
Sens	sensitivity
SMA	shape memory alloy
Spec	specificity
SPECT	single photon emission computed tomography
SPI	serial peripheral interface
SPSi	start point stiffness
succ	successor (child)
UART	universal asynchronous receiver-transmitter
USART	universal synchronous asynchronous receiver-transmitter
VLSI	very-large-scale-integration

Symbols

ΔP	change in applied pressure
$\Delta V / V$	relative change in the volume of the medium
$u(t)$	unit step function
$\frac{P_2}{P_1}$	ratio of power
$\frac{X_2}{X_1}$	ratio of force (current or voltage)
a	intercept (the output signal at zero input signal) or scalar constant or value of muscle activations or acceleration
A	cross-section area or state matrix
a_m	constant
b	slope (sensitivity) or linear damping coefficient
B	magnetic flux density or bulk modulus of elasticity or input matrix
c	compression
C	capacitance of a parallel-plate capacitor or pyroelectric coefficient or output matrix

$C(s)$	output Laplace transform
c_0	velocity of light in vacuum
d	distance between the plates in a capacitor or diameter
D	feed forward matrix or dimension
D_m	period of increase in stress graph
E	electric field or stiffness
E_{gland}	elastic modulus of gland
E_{fat}	elastic modulus of fat
E_{mass}	elastic modulus of mass
E_{skin}	elastic modulus of skin
F	force
f	number of one degree of freedom joints or nonlinear function or transfer function
F_{max}	maximum isometric force
f_s	frequency
$G(s)$	gain (ratio of the output Laplace transform divided by the input Laplace transform)
h	width or height
h/h_m	mass depth ratio
I	current or intensity of sound wave
J	optimization parameter
I_0	reference sound intensity
k_1	linear stiffness coefficient
k_2	cubic stiffness coefficient
l	length
L	inductance or self-inductance
$L[f(t)]$	Laplace transform
l_m	mass distance from reference point
l^{MT}	total length of the actuators
m	mass
M	degrees of freedom
M_H	torque about the hip joint
M_K	torque about the knee joint
mmf	magnetomotive force
MN	number of muscles
M_T	driving torque

n	number of links including a single ground link or number of quantization bits
N	number of turns in the coil or number of bit combinations or number of inputs
o	output
P_X	pressure of the sensor at position x
q	electric charge
q_i	axis
r	radius
R	reluctance of a magnetic field or resistance
R_H	Hall coefficient
$R(s)$	input Laplace transform
s	complex number
S	output
$S\ (\text{von Mises})_{\max}$	maximum von Mises stress
$S_{\exp}$	output of experiment
S_S	saturated value
$SupT$	supination torque
t_0	initial time
T_1	tight side tension
T_2	slack side tension
t	time or thickness or depth
T	temperature
T_d	decay time
T_e	effective tension
t_{int}	fat thickness
T_{off}	offset time of the input signal
T_{on}	onset time of the input signal
T_r	response time
T_s	sampling period taken at regular intervals
u	input or control vector
$u(t)$	unit step function
v	velocity
V	voltage
V_H	Hall voltage
V_L	voltage of inductance
ν_{mass}	Poisson's ratio of mass

$v[n]$	discrete time signal
$\nu_{\text{skin-fat-gland}}$	Poisson's ratio of skin, fat and gland
$v(t)$	analog signal
w	width
W	matrix of weights
w_i	weights associated with the inputs
x	state vector
$\dot{x}$	derivative of the state vector with respect to time
x_i	inputs
X	input or matrix of inputs
X_{exp}	input of experiment
X_1	linear input
X_0	particular input value
$x(t_0)$	initial conditions
X_{true}	true input
y	output vector

Greek Symbols

α	absorption
β	sound intensity level
ε	dielectric constant
ε_0	permittivity of free space in a capacitor
ε_r	relative permittivity or dielectric constant of the dielectric material
ϕ	flux
ρ_0	density
μ	permeability of a material
μ_0	magnetic permittivity of free space
μ_R	relative permeability of a material
ω	angular velocities
τ	torque exerted on the prosthetic ankle and knee
$(\ddot{\tau}_H)_{\text{exp.}}$	experimental calculated torque at the hip joint
$(\ddot{\tau}_K)_{\text{exp.}}$	experimental calculated torque at knee joint
θ	angle of ankle or knee
θ_e	balance angle
$\ddot{\theta}_H$	hip rotational accelerations
$\ddot{\theta}_K$	shank rotational accelerations

Index

F

G

H

CPSIA information can be obtained at www.ICGtesting.com
Printed in the USA
BVOW081942010312

284247BV00005B/2/P

9 780071 768962